Healthy Communities: New Partnerships for the Future of Public Health

Michael A. Stoto, Cynthia Abel, and Anne Dievler, *Editors*

A Report of the First Year of the
Committee on Public Health

INSTITUTE OF MEDICINE

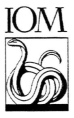

NATIONAL ACADEMY PRESS
Washington, D.C. 1996

INSTITUTE OF MEDICINE · 2101 Constitution Avenue, NW, · Washington, DC 20418

NOTICE: The project that is the subject of this report was approved by the Governing Board of the National Research Council, whose members are drawn from the councils of the National Academy of Sciences, the National Academy of Engineering, and the Institute of Medicine. The members of the committee responsible for this report were chosen for their special competencies and with regard for appropriate balance.

This report has been reviewed by a group other than the authors according to procedures approved by a Report Review Committee consisting of members of the National Academy of Sciences, the National Academy of Engineering, and the Institute of Medicine. The Institute of Medicine was chartered in 1970 by the National Academy of Sciences to enlist distinguished members of the appropriate professions in the examination of policy matters pertaining to the health of the public. In this, the Institute acts under both the Academy's 1863 congressional charter responsibility to be an adviser to the federal government and its own initiative in identifying issues of medical care, research, and education. Dr. Kenneth I. Shine is president of the Institute of Medicine.

Support for this project was provided by W. K. Kellogg Foundation, The Robert Wood Johnson Foundation, and by Grant Number H75/CCH311468-02 from the Centers for Disease Control and Prevention. The contents of this report reflect the views of the Committee on Public Health and are not necessarily those of the sponsors.

International Standard Book Number 0-309-05625-X

Additional copies of this report are available for sale from the National Academy Press, Box 285, 2101 Constitution Avenue, N.W., Washington, DC 20055. Call (800) 624-6242 or (202) 334-3313 (in the Washington metropolitan area), or visit the NAP's on-line bookstore at **http://www.nap.edu.**

Printed in the United States of America

The serpent has been a symbol of long life, healing, and knowledge among almost all cultures and religions since the beginning of recorded history. The image adopted as a logotype by the Institute of Medicine is based on a relief carving from ancient Greece, now held by the Staatlichemuseen in Berlin.

First Printing, December 1996   Fourth Printing, September 1997
Second Printing, April 1997   Fifth Printing, September 1998
Third Printing, July 1997   Sixth Printing, March 2000

COMMITTEE ON PUBLIC HEALTH

STUART BONDURANT* (*Cochair*), Interim Dean and Professor of Medicine, University of North Carolina School of Medicine, Chapel Hill

HUGH H. TILSON (*Cochair*), Professor of Epidemiology and Health Policy, University of North Carolina School of Public Health, Chapel Hill

MARGARET A. HAMBURG,* Health Commissioner, New York City Department of Health

JOHN LUMPKIN, Director, Illinois Department of Public Health, Springfield

ROBERT B. WALLACE, Professor of Preventive and Internal Medicine and Director, Cancer Center, University of Iowa

Institute of Medicine Staff

MICHAEL A. STOTO, Director, Division of Health Promotion and Disease Prevention

CYNTHIA ABEL, Program Officer

DONNA THOMPSON, Division Assistant

ANNE DIEVLER, Consultant

MONA BRINEGAR, Financial Associate (through July 1995)

SHARON GALLOWAY, Financial Associate (after September 1995)

Liaison Panel to the Committee on Public Health

EDWARD L. BAKER, Director, Public Health Practice Program Office, Centers for Disease Control and Prevention, Atlanta, Ga.

STEVE BOEDIGHEIMER, Deputy Director, Division of Public Health, Delaware Health and Social Services, Dover

JO IVEY BOUFFORD, Principal Deputy Assistant Secretary for Health, U.S. Public Health Service, Department of Health and Human Services, Washington, D.C.

E. RICHARD BROWN, Professor of Public Health, School of Public Health and Director, Center for Health Policy Research, University of California, Los Angeles

THOMAS A. BRUCE, Program Director, W.K. Kellogg Foundation, Battle Creek, Mich.

CASWELL A. EVANS, JR.,* Assistant Director of Health Services, Director, Public Health Programs and Services, County of Los Angeles, Department of Health Services

---

*Institute of Medicine member.

Preface

In 1988, after extensive review of data, interviews, forums, and analyses, the Institute of Medicine (IOM) released a landmark report, *The Future of Public Health*. While this report raised questions about many aspects of public health as it was practiced at the time, it also found much to commend. Its primary impact was setting forth a "vision" for public health, including the mission and substance of governmental public health agencies, an organizational framework, and specific recommendations. *The Future of Public Health* also served as a catalyst for change in the public health system, and the response to the report was wide ranging, varied, and extensive. During the years since *The Future of Public Health* was released, there has been a significant strengthening of practice by governmental public health agencies in many respects.

Almost a decade after the committee that wrote *The Future of Public Health* was created, the IOM established the Committee on Public Health to review the progress that has been made since the release of *The Future of Public Health* and to address selected areas that have experienced substantial changes. To assist the committee in its efforts, the IOM also identified a liaison panel of people from government, academia, industry, and citizen and other private-sector groups to help identify emerging issues and to facilitate an informed dialogue on current issues in public health. This group was called the Public Health Roundtable.

The discussions initiated by the Committee on Public Health were richly substantive and allowed its members to address, fundamental issues in public health that were not being dealt with in other settings. Over a nine-month period, the committee held three meetings focused on (1) progress toward achieving the recommendations presented in *The Future of Public Health*, (2) the relationship between public health agencies and managed care organizations, and (3) the emerging role of the public health agency in the community. These discussions revealed that although they are making gains on some fronts and losing ground on others, public health agencies are alive and well. The discussions also revealed an astonishing array of activities being carried out in response to *The Future of Public Health*.

The substance of this report is drawn from the committee's discussions and other related IOM projects, but the conclusions presented in this report are those of the Committee on Public Health. The material in the text boxes is drawn from presentations at committee meetings and from members of the liaison panel. These boxes are intended to give the reader a sense of the committee's discussions but do not necessarily represent a consensus of the committee.

During its first year, the Committee on Public Health was able to address only some of the many issues in public health today. In the course of its deliberations, the committee encountered evidence that many of the problems identified in *The Future of Public Health* were still with us. In light of these limitations, the committee's first-year report does not aim to replace *The Future of Public Health*, but rather to supplement and update it in two critical areas: the relationship between public health agencies and the public's health and managed care, and the role of the public health agency in the community. The committee recognizes that not all local public health agencies are currently dealing with the issues covered in the report, but we believe that the report should be useful to all agencies as they think about how to approach these issues in the future.

As cochairs of the Committee on Public Health, we gratefully acknowledge the contributions of the committee, the Public Health Roundtable, and the many people (listed in the appendixes) with whom we met during the course of our work. We would like to thank Anne Dievler, who worked with IOM staff members in drafting several sections of the report and Michael Edington, who provided excellent editorial skills. We would like to give special thanks to the staff for this project, Michael Stoto, Cynthia Abel, and Donna Thompson, for their tireless efforts to organize and synthesize the committee's activities.

Stuart Bondurant, *Cochair*
Hugh Tilson, *Cochair*

Contents

Executive Summary

The Future of Public Health, issued in 1988, set forth a vision of public health and a specific role for the governmental public health agency within that vision, including the mission and content of public health, and an organizational framework. In the eight years since the report was released, there has been a significant strengthening of practice in governmental public health agencies and other settings. Substantial social, demographic, and technological changes in recent years, however, have made it necessary to reexamine governmental public health agencies' efforts to improve the public's health. Drawing on the activities and discussions initiated by the Institute of Medicine (IOM) Committee on Public Health, the current report addresses two critical public health issues that can greatly influence the opportunity for our public to be healthy as the United States enters a new century—(1) the relationship between public health agencies and managed care organizations, and (2) the role of the public health agency in the community—and their implications for the broader issues raised in *The Future of Public Health*.

The committee's analysis, presented in this report, reaffirmed the understanding of public health professionals and health scientists that **the public's health depends on the interaction of many factors; thus, the health of a community is a shared responsibility of many entities, organizations, and interests in the community, including health service delivery organizations, public health agencies, other public and private entities, and the people of a community. Within this context of shared responsibility, specific entities should identify, and be held accountable for, the actions they can take to contribute toward the community's health.** As a result of this understanding,

1

the committee focused its report on how governmental public health agencies, especially at the state and local level, can develop partnerships with managed care organizations for the delivery of personal and population-based health services and with public and private community organizations to deal with broader concerns to advance the health of the community. Developing these partnerships, the committee believes, will be critical for advancing the health of the public and of communities in the future.

PUBLIC HEALTH AND MANAGED CARE

There has been substantial growth in organized health care delivery systems (which include managed care organizations) in recent years, and these developments have important implications for the health of the public. Managed care organizations are systems that are under the management of a single entity that (a) insures members, (b) furnishes covered benefits through a defined network of participating providers, and (c) manages the health care practices of participating providers. In the discussions initiated by the Public Health Committee, proponents of managed care have argued that its goals and tools are consistent with public health. Many public health professionals, on the other hand, have also expressed concerns about managed care organizations' motives and ability to deliver on their promises. The committee's view, as developed in this section, is that if the proper kinds of partnerships between managed care organizations and governmental public health departments are developed, managed care can indeed make an important contribution to improving the health of the public.

The proliferation of organized health care delivery systems, which continue to provide care for an increasing number of Americans, has made it possible in some locales for governmental public health agencies to assure the provision of personal health services (which involve a one-to-one interaction between patient and provider) entirely within the private sector. How many elements of public health services private organizations can or should subsume remains unclear, but the number could be considerable. Providing care for the uninsured, however, remains a challenge; governmental public health departments will be ill prepared and inadequately funded to do so if no other personal services are being provided.

In order to ensure that partnerships between governmental public health agencies and managed care organizations work effectively toward improving the health of the public, the committee reiterates *The Future of Public Health* recommendation that **the function of local public health agencies should include an "assurance that high-quality services, including personal health services, needed for the protection of public health in the community are available and**

accessible to all persons. . . ." This assurance function can be carried out "by encouraging other entities (private or public sector), by requiring such actions through regulation, or by providing services directly." Public health agencies can only exercise this responsibility if they are adequately staffed, equipped, and funded for this complex and demanding task and have appropriate relationships with health service providers. These activities should not be undertaken at the expense of existing essential public health services. Particular concerns arise when health departments have a dual role: direct provision of personal health services to some people and regulating private entities providing similar services to others. To improve the efficiency of all health systems, **health agencies and organized health delivery systems, in conjunction with other community stakeholders, must reach agreement on their proper roles and responsibilities, which will vary by locale.** Successful models of the integration of public health and managed care and of joint approaches to policy development do exist and need to be studied and tested more broadly.

Most public health agencies do not currently have the full statutory and regulatory authority to ensure the accountability of the organized health delivery systems to the public. In the current regulatory structure, health care delivery systems are often regulated by insurance commissions that focus on fiscal integrity rather than on health. State Medicaid agencies, usually separate from public health departments, also typically focus on fiscal rather than medical accountability dimensions, except in states that have a quality initiative. Recognizing the clear need for financial oversight, **governmental public health agencies should increase their ability to oversee health care providers, with the goal of becoming coequal partners with insurance regulators and state Medicaid agencies, to ensure that the public's health is addressed in the regulation of public and private health care delivery systems.** In many states, additional legislative authority will be needed before public health agencies can take on this role. This approach requires population-based health outcome and performance standards that can be monitored, and public health agencies should be a major contributor to the development and monitoring of these standards.

The functions described in this report cannot be undertaken without properly trained professionals available to all communities. Thus, **public health professionals should be trained to work with health services organizations to ensure quality personal health services in a community, as an essential element in providing for the health of the public.** In addition, **public health agencies should actively participate with organizations such as state health professions boards, medical schools, and accrediting bodies in planning and policy development.**

PUBLIC HEALTH AND THE COMMUNITY

In its discussions with community group representatives and public health officials, the committee heard of many innovative and effective approaches to community partnerships and collaboration that are consistent with widespread themes regarding community development and "reinventing government." Broader application and further development of these new approaches to collaboration within government (with legislators, boards of health, and nonhealth agencies) and with community partners to achieve public health goals should be encouraged.

Shared responsibility, however, requires careful management. **The governmental public health agency in each community needs to be capable of identifying and working with all of the entities that influence a community's health, especially those that are not directly health related. This function must be undertaken by public health agencies that understand the interactions of the full range of factors that influence the community's health.** To address this, a companion IOM report proposes a "community health improvement process" that draws on performance monitoring concepts, an understanding of community development, and the role of public health consistent with the Committee on Public Health's discussions (IOM, in press). **Public health professionals who must work with a community to improve its own health need to be trained and their roles need to be upgraded or enhanced.**

The committee's discussions showed that **many functions essential to the public's health, such as immunizations and health education, can and are being performed by either public or private entities, depending on the historical context, community resources, and political dynamics of a particular area. Some functions, however, such as environmental regulation and enforcement of public health laws, must remain the responsibility of governmental public health agencies.** There also needs to be a resource in each community to ensure that the health impact of multiple interventions in the community are understood and addressed. This remains an ideal function for governmental public health agencies and should not be delegated. Thus, the committee reasserts the critical findings of *The Future of Public Health* that **governmental public health agencies have a unique function in the community: "to see to it that vital elements are in place and that the [public health] mission is adequately addressed." These elements include assessment, policy development, and assurance.** For a governmental agency to execute this responsibility effectively, there must be explicit legal authority, as well as health goals and functions, that the public understands and demands. A fundamental building block for this new approach to governance is public trust. With trust in public institutions at risk or at low levels in many communities, governmental public health agencies must find ways to improve their openness and their communication with the public to maintain and increase their trustworthiness.

REVISITING *THE FUTURE OF PUBLIC HEALTH*

Through its analysis of the interactions between managed care organizations and governmental public health agencies and the role of public health agencies to enhance the health of the community, and through its discussions about the many responses to *The Future of Public Health*, the committee found that the constructs of the mission and substance for public health agencies envisioned in that report have been extraordinarily useful in revitalizing the infrastructure and rebuilding the system of public health at all levels of government in the United States and continue to be viewed as the fundamental building blocks for the future. However, although clear progress has been made, some of the recommendations of that report have not yet been implemented. In light of this, the committee's analysis shows that **the concepts in *The Future of Public Health* remain vital and essential to current and future efforts to energize and focus the efforts of public health. These concepts need to be advanced, applied, and taught to all health professionals.**

The committee also found that **the concepts of assessment, policy development, and assurance**, while useful in the public health community itself, have been difficult to translate into effective messages for key stakeholders, including elected officials and community groups. These concepts **need to be translated into a vernacular that these groups can understand.**

In conclusion, the committee found that the public health enterprise in the United States, as embodied in governmental public health agencies, is necessarily diverse in organization and function, but operates within the common framework set out in *The Future of Public Health*. The committee's discussions, however, revealed continuing evidence of inadequate support for governmental public health agencies in many communities. Now, as nearly a decade before, **society must reinvest in governmental public health agencies, with resources, commitments, and contributions from government, private and non-profit sectors, and substantial legal authorities, if the public's health is to improve.**
The partnerships that are the focus of this report—between governmental public health agencies and managed care organizations, and between public health and the community—can provide both political support and a vehicle for this reinvestment.

Introduction

The Future of Public Health set forth a vision for the public's health and the specific role for the governmental public health agency in that vision, including the mission and substance of public health and an organizational framework. In this perspective, the public's health is a societal priority and goal, to be achieved by governmental public health agencies and other public and private entities in the community. Public health is also a perspective and a profession, both of which focus on improving the health of the public.

Specifically, *The Future of Public Health* stated that the mission of public health agencies is "fulfilling society's interest in assuring conditions in which people can be healthy. Its aim is to generate organized community effort to address the public interest in health by applying scientific and technical knowledge to prevent disease and promote health. The mission of public health is addressed by private organizations and individuals as well as by public agencies. But the governmental public health agency has a unique function: to see to it that vital elements are in place and that the mission is adequately addressed." *The Future of Public Health*, expressed the basic governmental responsibility for the people's health as assuring a substantive core of activities, assuring adequacy of means and methods, establishing objectives, and providing guarantees in an ideal health system, the substance of basic services will entail adequate personal health care for all members of the community, education of the community-at-large, the control of communicable disease, and the control of environmental hazards—biological, chemical, social, and physical (IOM, 1988).

The report defined the three core functions of public health as:

1. Assessment—"Every public health agency [should] regularly and systematically collect, assemble, analyze, and make available information on the health of the community, including statistics on health status, community health needs, and epidemiologic and other studies of health problems. Not every agency is large enough to conduct these activities directly; intergovernmental and interagency cooperation is essential. Nevertheless each agency bears the responsibility for seeing that the assessment function is fulfilled. This basic function of public health cannot be delegated."

2. Policy development—"Every public health agency [should] exercise its responsibility to serve the public interest in the development of comprehensive public health policies by promoting use of the scientific knowledge base in decision-making about public health and by leading in developing public health policy. Agencies must take a strategic approach, developed on the basis of a positive appreciation for the democratic political process."

3. Assurance—"Public health agencies [should] assure their constituents that services necessary to achieve agreed upon goals are provided, by either encouraging actions by other entities (private or public sector), by requiring such action through regulation, or by providing services directly. . . . Public health agenc[ies should] involve key policymakers and the general public in determining a set of high-priority personal and communitywide health services that governments will guarantee to every member of the community. This guarantee should include subsidization or direct provision of high-priority personal health services for those unable to afford them" (IOM, 1988).

In the eight years since this report was released, there has been a significant strengthening of practice in governmental public health agencies and other settings. Substantial social, demographic, and technological changes in recent years (Brownson and Kreuter, in press), however, have made it necessary to reexamine governmental public health agencies' efforts to improve the public's health.

Building upon the concepts of assessment, assurance, and policy development contained in *The Future of Public Health*, a group of leading public health organizations (Public Health Functions Steering Committee, 1994[1]) adopted a

---

[1] Members of the Public Health Functions Steering Committee include: American Public Health Association; Association of State and Territorial Health Officials; National Association of County and City Health Officials; Institute of Medicine, National Academy of Sciences; Association of Schools of Public Health; Public Health Foundation; National Association of State Alcohol and Drug Abuse Directors; and the

vision of public health as "healthy people in healthy communities," six public health goals, and ten essential public health services. The six public health goals are to: (1) prevent epidemics and the spread of disease, (2) protect against environmental hazards, (3) prevent injuries, (4) promote and encourage healthy behaviors, (5) respond to disasters and assist communities in recovery, and (6) assure the quality and accessibility of health services.

The ten essential public health services are to:

1. monitor health status to identify community health problems;
2. diagnose and investigate health problems and health hazards in the community;
3. inform, educate, and empower people about health issues;
4. mobilize community partnerships to identify and solve health problems;
5. develop policies and plans that support individual and community health efforts;
6. enforce laws and regulations that protect health and ensure safety;
7. link people to needed personal health services and ensure the provision of health care when it is otherwise unavailable;
8. ensure the availability of a competent public health and personal health care workforce;
9. evaluate effectiveness, accessibility, and quality of personal and population-based health services; and
10. research new insights and innovative solutions to health problems.

These essential public health services were used to describe public health more readily to external audiences and constituencies and played an important role in defining public health during the 1993–1994 health care reform debate (Turnock and Handler, 1995).

FACTORS AFFECTING PUBLIC HEALTH

We live in a complexly, interconnected global society in which there are many threats to, and opportunities to improve, the public's health. In recent years, we have witnessed the emergence or reemergence of infectious diseases such as hanta virus, cryptosporidiosis, *Escherichia. coli* O157, and Ebola virus (Gordon et

---

U.S. Public Health Service (Centers for Disease Control and Prevention, Health Resources and Services Administration, Office of the Assistant Secretary for Health, Substance Abuse and Mental Health Services Administration, Agency for Health Care Policy and Research, Indian Health Services, and Food and Drug Administration).

al., 1996). In the late 1980s and early 1990s, tuberculosis made a comeback in cities across the United States, with many drug-resistant cases arising (OTA, 1993; Gittler, 1994), and outbreaks of childhood diseases such as measles and mumps appeared among poor inner city children (Atkinson et al., 1992; Kelley et al., 1993; Vivier et al., 1994). The number of human immunodeficiency virus/ acquired immunodeficiency syndrome (HIV/AIDS) cases has surpassed 500,000 in the United States, and among persons aged 25–44 years, HIV infection is the leading cause of death in men and the third-leading cause in women (CDC, 1995a).

Despite these outbreaks, which remain important, the 20th century has seen a shift in the major causes of death from infectious to chronic diseases, and behavioral risk factors have increased in importance. Behavior-related factors such as use of tobacco, alcohol, illicit drugs, firearms, and motor vehicles, as well as diet, activity patterns, and sexual behavior, are responsible for nearly half of the deaths in the United States and substantial amounts of disability (McGinnis and Foege, 1993). Reflecting these realities, behavior and lifestyle interventions are highlighted, for instance, in *Healthy People 2000: National Health Promotion and Disease Prevention Objectives* (DHHS, 1991), with attention paid not only to the behaviors themselves but also to lifestyle more generally and to the context and social circumstances that influence individual behavior.

Consistent with the development of these trends, public health professionals have come to realize that health is a dynamic state that is influenced by many internal and external process, and that embraces well-being—physical, mental, and emotional health. For both individuals and populations, health improvement depends not only on medical care but also on other factors including individual behavior, genetic makeup, and social and economic conditions for individuals and communities. The Field Model, as described by Evans and Stoddart (1994), presents these multiple determinants of health in a dynamic relationship. A wide range of actors, many of whose roles are not within the traditional domain of health activities, have an effect on and a stake in a community's health (Patrick and Wickizer, 1995). The Field Model suggests a variety of public and private entities in the community that, through their actions, could influence the community's health. As communities try to address their health issues in a comprehensive manner, everyone involved will need to sort out their roles and responsibilities. They also should participate in the process of "community-wide social change" that is needed to improve health (Green and Kreuter, 1990).

As the public health community was coming to appreciate these ideas about the root determinants of health, other concerns about the high and rising costs of health care, the lack of geographical and economic access to health services for many, and questions about the quality and timeliness of the care provided led to many governmental and private attempts to alter the organization, delivery, and funding of health care. Foremost among these attempts in the past decade has been the growth in organized health care delivery systems, including managed care, and the size of the organizations that deliver it (Gabel et al., 1994; Robinson, 1996). However, the implications of these changes in the mode of service delivery and funding for public health agencies are uncertain. Has access for disadvantaged populations improved or worsened? Can public health agencies delegate or contract their clinical health promotion and disease prevention and control programs to emerging health care organizations? If they can, can the quality and effectiveness of such programs be assured? Is ensuring adequate clinical health care for all an important public health priority?

As the health system has changed, so too has the political landscape. Although Americans have been skeptical of government since the founding of this country, in recent years there has been a growing mistrust of government, government institutions, and politics (Dionne, 1991; La Porte and Metlay, 1996; *Washington Post*, 1996). Although distrust of government has received considerable attention, trust in other institutions such as the press, religious institutions, banking, and business has also been challenged. Related to this lack of confidence in government, or perhaps in response to it, is a decided shift in responsibility from the federal government to state and local levels. Furthermore, there has been a growing movement to "reinvent government," including making it more decentralized, responsive to clients or "customers," community-oriented, and entrepreneurial by employing performance monitoring and outcomes standards (Osborne and Gaebler, 1992). In many communities, public health functions previously performed directly by government employees are being carried out by employees of private organizations. As a result, the opportunities for public-private partnerships are greater than ever before.

SUMMARY AND ORGANIZATION OF THIS REPORT

In summary, the discussions initiated by the Committee on Public Health have suggested that three key forces shaping public health are (1) the rise of organized health care delivery systems, including managed care; (2) the changing role and public expectations of government; and (3) the increasing involvement and mobilization of communities in matters pertaining to their own health. Drawing on the committee's activities and discussions, this report addresses two critical public health issues in the United States as it enters a new century—the relationship between public health and managed care, and the role of the public health agency in the community—and their implications for the broader infrastructure and capacity issues raised in *The Future of Public Health*.

The committee's analysis, presented in this report, reaffirmed the understanding of public health professionals and health scientists that **the public's health depends on the interaction of many factors; thus, the health of a community is a shared responsibility of many entities, organizations, and interests in the community, including health service delivery organizations, public health agencies, other public and private entities, and the people of a community. Within this context of shared responsibility, specific entities should identify, and be held accountable for, the actions they can take to contribute toward the community's health.** As a result of this understanding, the committee focused its report on how governmental public health agencies, especially at the state and local levels, can develop partnerships with managed care organizations to deliver personal and population-based health services and with public and private community organizations to deal with broader concerns to advance the health of the community. Developing these partnerships, the committee believes, will be critical for advancing the health of the public and of communities in the future.

Public Health and Managed Care

In the past decade, there has been substantial growth in organized health care delivery systems in most parts of the United States. Managed care organizations, the most common form of these systems, can be defined as "any system that is under the management of a single entity that (1) insures members—either by itself or through an intermediary, (2) furnishes covered benefits through a defined network of participating providers, and (3) manages the health care practices of participating providers" (Rosenbaum and Richards, 1996).

Public health practice is sometimes thought of as separate from, or complementary to, the delivery of personal health services. A more helpful distinction is between personal health services and community interventions. Personal health services involve a one-to-one interaction between a provider and a patient (IOM, 1993). Personal health services are delivered primarily by private-sector organizations, but in many communities, governmental health departments provide many of these services, especially for disadvantaged populations. Community interventions aim to alter the social or physical environment to change one or more health-related behaviors or to directly reduce the risk of causing a health problem. Community-based services are usually carried out by public health agencies, other government agencies, or community-based voluntary organizations. The provision of personal health services per se, even if they are delivered in the community rather than in health care settings, is not a community intervention. Outreach or community-based activities intended to improve access to personal health services or their utilization, however, are included. Public health agencies are often challenged to provide both types of services, but community organizations frequently help the public health agency

13

achieve a public health objective in a community (Box 1). Private health service organizations sometimes sponsor outreach activities such as mass screening and health fairs (at times with commercial interests), with and without a public health agency's involvement.

BOX 1. Overcoming Barriers to Immunization: An Example for Public Health

In 1992 the 16,000 members of the Florida District of Kiwanis International formed a partnership with the Department of Health and Rehabilitative Services' (HRS's) State Health Office Immunization Program to help increase immunization levels in the preschool population. As part of their "Young Children: Priority One" major initiative, the Florida District Kiwanis made an eight-year commitment to be lead volunteer agency assisting in implementing Florida's Immunization Action Plan. This plan provides objectives to raise the immunization rates of Florida's two-year-olds to 90% by the year 2000. At the time of the formation of the partnership, only 63% of Florida's two-year-olds were up to date with their immunizations. Since the HRS-Kiwanis partnership was formed four years ago, the immunization levels have increased by 27%.

The Kiwanis have donated many thousands of volunteer hours in immunization clinics and have organized coalitions, recruited other community groups, and purchased computer equipment, vans, and educational materials. With the Kiwanis's help, Florida's 67 county public health units have increased their clinic hours, opened new clinic sites, extended service times and added locations, arranged transportation services for low-income clients, and coordinated services with other agencies to reach more children. Because of this partnership, more of Florida's young children are protected against vaccine-preventable diseases now than at any other time in the state's history. The 1995 Survey of Immunization Levels in the two-year-old population indicated that an unprecedented 80% of Florida's two-year-olds are immunized. Much of the increase can be attributed to the Kiwanis's leadership in volunteer efforts.

This partnership has helped reduce the dangers that exist when society fails to immunize its children. For example, the number of measles cases in Florida had nearly doubled, from 322 cases in 1989 to 603 cases in 1990. Two of the cases occurred among unvaccinated preschool children. In 1995, there were 14 confirmed measles cases in Florida. Through this partnership, the Kiwanis, the county public health units, and the immunization program office have set an example that demonstrates the positive benefits that result when a community-based partnership works together to donate time, energy, and resources to improve the health of Florida's children.

SOURCE: Based on information provided by Charles Mahan, Dean of the University of South Florida College of Public Health (former director, Florida State Department of Health and Rehabilitative Services), 1996.

An estimated 90 million insured Americans are enrolled in managed care plans, including more than 25% of Medicaid beneficiaries and 10% of Medicare beneficiaries (Rosenbaum and Richards, 1996). Most of the growth in enrollment has occurred in recent years. Between 1988 and 1993, the percentage of employees enrolled in a managed care plan increased from 29% to 51% (Gabel et al., 1994). In the Medicaid program, the growth has been even more dramatic as states have requested waivers from the Health Care Financing Administration (HCFA) to shift their Medicaid populations into managed care arrangements. Between 1993 and 1994, the number of Medicaid beneficiaries in managed care increased by 63%, from 4.8 million to 7.8 million (Kaiser Commission, 1995). The factors contributing to the growth in managed care are the rising costs of personal health care and an interest among employers to find ways to control providers and, therefore, to control costs (Rosenbaum and Richards, 1996). States have also used managed care arrangements as a way of containing spiraling costs in the Medicaid program and of trying to improve access to care (Kaiser Commission, 1995).

STRENGTHS AND WEAKNESSES OF MANAGED CARE FOR PUBLIC HEALTH

Managed care offers opportunities for public health (CDC and GHAA, n.d.; Baker et al., 1994; HRSA, n.d.) but it also poses challenges. In the discussions initiated by the Public Health Committee, proponents of managed care have argued that its goals and tools are consistent with public health. Many public health professionals, on the other hand, have also indicated concern about managed care organizations' motives and ability to deliver on their promises. The committee's view, as developed in this section, is that if the proper kinds of partnerships between managed care organizations and governmental public health departments are developed, managed care can indeed make an important contribution to improving the health of the public.

Accountability, Responsibility, and Quality

Because it is responsible for delivering care to a defined group of enrollees, managed care makes possible, for the first time, accountability in terms of quality of care for populations, including access to care and health outcomes. This is possible because managed care organizations can monitor the health outcomes of enrollees and examine their use of services. However, this is not regularly done. Some managed care organizations, especially large staff-model managed care organizations, are using their data systems to track the health of their enrollees, but many managed care organizations do not collect the types of information needed for surveillance and epidemiologic studies. There have been a number of attempts to assess the quality of care offered by managed care organizations. The National Committee for Quality Assurance (NCQA), which accredits managed care organizations, has developed the Health Plan Employer Data and Information Set (HEDIS), a set of performance measures for managed care organizations designed to meet employers' and government purchasers' needs for information about the value of services they purchase and to systematize the measurement process (NCQA, 1993).

The data systems maintained by some managed care organizations are an important tool for improving performance and maintaining accountability, and simply by having performance monitoring systems, these organizations compare favorably with fee-for-service delivery systems or indemnity insurance companies that typically have no data with which to monitor performance. The committee heard of instances in which a managed care organization's performance—in terms of provision of preventive services, for example—was criticized based on the organization's own data, with the implicit assumption that other providers do better. Such assumptions may well be incorrect and are unfair because they cannot be checked unless the other providers have appropriate data systems. Experience suggests that performance monitoring as a basis for punishing those who are not producing as expected is not an effective way to alter behavior and improve outcomes. Rather, performance monitoring should be used to encourage productive action and broad collaboration (Berwick, 1989; IOM, in press).

Population Orientation and Prevention

Managed care's responsibility for a defined population gives it an interest in promoting health and preventing disease in that population, which is the mission of public health. Both managed care organizations and governmental public health agencies have a philosophical emphasis on promoting health and preventing disease. Both address prevention and health promotion in a defined population. However, in actual practice, some managed care organizations seem more concerned about efficiency and controlling short-run costs than about prevention or the health status of their members. Governmental public health agencies have a geographic perspective and are accountable to the people within their jurisdiction while many managed care organizations focus on their current enrollees, an ever-changing group, who may only be a subset of the population. Committee discussions suggested that in the long term, it is important for managed care organizations to think more broadly and to promote health in the whole community because anyone may be their enrollee in the future (Box 2). In a capitated system with limited turnover, some prevention activities might result in larger future profit margins. Unlike public health agencies, managed care organizations are primarily accountable to purchasers, subscribing employers, large groups of payers, and ultimately their stockholders or trustees. As managed care organizations respond to public demands for accountability, more should find ways to measure the quality of services they provide. A focus on health outcomes and prevention objectives, as some organizations which have adopted HEDIS and other performance measures have done, would help.

BOX 2. Group Health Cooperative of Puget Sound

Group Health Cooperative of Puget Sound is a large, nonprofit health maintenance organization (HMO) that was established in 1947. It has approximately 540,000 enrollees, of whom about 80,000–90,000 are enrolled in the Medicare and Medicaid Basic Health Plan. The cooperative has been involved in community-based health for more than 50 years. Its public health focus grew out of 10 years of involvement with public health in community issues and priorities such as AIDS prevention.

In 1992, Group Health adopted a vision statement that calls for delivery of quality health care to the whole community, not just its enrolled population. They also adopted a set of community service principles to recognize the work that Group Health had been doing in the community in the area of health promotion and disease prevention. They currently focus their attention on four areas: (1) childhood immunization, (2) the reduction of infant mortality, (3) health care for homeless families, and (4) the reduction and prevention of interpersonal violence. In their community-based programs, Group Health has gone beyond just providing immunization and preventive clinical services to issues that deal with changing social norms, such as violence and alcohol abuse. Group Health is also working with the State of Washington on surveillance issues to improve their performance measurements and develop more integrated information systems.

Group Health considered several factors in implementing its community programs. Improving community health in general is expected to lead to improved health for the members of Group Health as well. Involvement in community-based programs also helps Group Health compete for contracts with large employer groups and with Medicaid and Medicare populations. In addition, community service programs help to encourage innovative approaches to providing services to the patient population.

SOURCE: Based on a presentation by William Berry, director, Center for Health Promotion, Group Health Cooperative of Puget Sound, at the February 22, 1996, meeting of the Public Health Committee.

Personal Health Services for Vulnerable Populations

As managed care organizations enroll increasing numbers of people from disadvantaged groups, the biggest challenge for public health agencies is in the area of providing personal health services for poor and vulnerable populations. Public health agencies, primarily at the local level, have played an important role in providing health care services to both Medicaid-eligible and uninsured and underinsured population groups. For example, they provide maternal and child health services, sexually transmitted disease (STD) services, and tuberculosis services. For certain services, issues of expertise or confidentiality would suggest that public health agencies are the appropriate entities to continue to provide these services (Frieden et al., 1995; IOM 1996), so local public health agencies must maintain this capacity. As more states shift their Medicaid enrollees into managed care, public health agencies have the option of trying to obtain contracts with managed care organizations, but many are ill-equipped to compete for and negotiate with health plans (Lipson and Naierman, 1996). Many issues of language, culture, tradition, class, race, and ethnicity need to be taken into account when providing services to especially vulnerable populations. Perhaps the most serious aspect of this problem is providing services to those who are covered by neither insurance nor Medicaid and who are especially vulnerable.

As many cities and counties move to privatize public hospitals, which have traditionally served vulnerable populations, they will have to consider whether and how managed care organizations fill this role and how the delivery of care to the underinsured and uninsured will continue. Individuals who are eligible for Medicaid but unfamiliar with managed care organizations may not understand how to access needed services. A strategy of partnering with both governmental public health agencies and community-based organizations, which have the skills and experience needed to work effectively with these vulnerable populations, could strengthen the entire health system's response to the needs of these special populations.

Many state Medicaid agencies do not have the management skills to monitor the performance of managed care organizations or to write appropriate contracts with these organizations (Box 3). Competitive cost-cutting pressures coupled with vulnerable populations may result in opportunities for health care plans or providers to take advantage of poor patients. The problem of turnover of patient population as enrollees lose and regain their eligibility for Medicaid also contributes to serious problems of continuity of care.

BOX 3. Medicaid Managed Care

The move toward managed care for Medicaid patients offers promise for improving health outcomes and solving potential problems. The promise is due to the shift inherent in managed care toward interest in the health of defined populations. This facilitates the use of public health assessment tools (e.g., epidemiology), strategic thinking about efficient ways to improve the health of populations, and opportunities to undertake activities focused on disease prevention.

Problems that may occur during this transition to Medicaid managed care include (1) personal health services traditionally carried out by public health departments (i.e., prenatal care, immunization services, family planning and sexually transmitted disease [STD] clinics, and Early and Periodic Screening, Diagnosis, and Treatment [EPSDT]) will not be completely transferred to a managed care organization; (2) poor people who are eligible for Medicaid but are unfamiliar with managed care organizations may not understand how to access needed service; (3) many state Medicaid agencies do not have the management skills to monitor the performance of managed care organizations or to write appropriate contracts with them; and (4) competitive cost-cutting pressures coupled with vulnerable populations and weak oversight may result in some unscrupulous health care providers taking advantage of poor patients.

There is a growing realization that managed care organizations need the expertise and authority of public health agencies to undertake community-based interventions and perform outreach services that are necessary for maintaining the health of the populations for which they are responsible. Public health services are also necessary in cases in which confidentiality is an issue, such as at STD or family planning clinics.

Many public health professionals now provide personal health services, often in community-based categorical public health clinics. Such services are the type that managed care organizations should be able to handle, and therefore, once they are trasferrred, there will be less of a need for health professionals with the same skills in public health departments. There will be an increased need in both public health departments and managed care organizations for people with public health assessment skills and health care management skills.

SOURCE: Presentations to the Institute of Medicine (IOM) Board on Health Promotion and Disease Prevention and the National Research Council/IOM Board on Children and Families in joint session on June 15, 1995.

DEFINING ROLES AND RESPONSIBILITIES

Given the challenges involved in the transition to managed care, it will be important for each community to define the roles and responsibilities of governmental public health agencies and managed care organizations in improving health. Depending on local conditions, public health agencies can play a variety of roles, from serving in an advisory or regulatory capacity to obtaining contracts to provide services. Managed care organizations can play a role in health promotion and disease prevention, disease surveillance, and promoting quality. The IOM report *The Hidden Epidemic: Confronting Sexually Transmitted Diseases* (1996), illustrates the opportunities and problems in the relationship between health department and managed care organizations in one area (Box 4). Two recent reports (CDC and GHAA, n.d.; Joint Council, 1996) identify a variety of approaches to collaboration. More generally, a new joint initiative of the American Medical Association and the American Public Health Association is exploring new ways that medicine and public health can collaborate to improve health and health care in the United States (Reiser, 1996).

BOX 4. IOM Committee on the Prevention and Control of Sexually Transmitted Diseases (STDs)

The Institute of Medicine (IOM) Committee on the Prevention and Control of STDs held a workshop on November 8, 1995, to examine the role of managed care in STD prevention and control. The national movement toward managed care coupled with limited public funds for health programs will have a significant impact on the delivery of services provided by public health agencies, especially those that involve many providers and intervention points such as STD prevention and control.

There are many opportunities and challenges for managed care to address STD issues effectively. Strengths of managed care organizations that are particularly appropriate for this role include (1) a population-based focus (i.e., group and staff models track disease and health trends for a population), (2) the ability to coordinate and integrate STD services into primary care, and (3) accountability to purchasers of health services.

Increasingly, managed care organizations are enrolling Medicaid populations whose health care used to be provided by local public health departments. In some states, Medicaid revenues have been a major source of funding for public health clinical services. The absence of the revenues becomes a problem for local health departments as well as for community-based health clinics that have been providing services. Nevertheless, local health departments report that many persons with health insurance continue to use public health clinics, local health department STD clinics, or other clinics outside of their health plan for STD-related services.

SOURCE: Presentation by Richard Brown, member of the IOM Committee on the Prevention and Control of STDs, at the February 22, 1996, meeting of the Public Health Committee; IOM (1996).

Roles for Public Health Agencies

With their potentially extensive knowledge of the community and its depth and breadth of experience in fields such as epidemiology and injury prevention, governmental public health agencies can play an important role with managed care organizations. *The Future of Public Health's* analysis implies that public health departments should work with managed care organizations, in the public interest, as part of their assessment and assurance mandate. Their role can include everything from offering advice about data and information systems, to developing training and education programs, even to fostering an advocacy role (Box 5). In particular, governmental public health agencies can:

• provide *information* about the health status, risks, and determinants of communities served by managed care organizations, which is vital for raising awareness and setting priorities even if the jurisdictions of the health agencies do not correspond exactly to the population covered by the managed care organizations;
• participate with managed care organizations in *planning and policy development* related to voluntary collaborative actions or regulatory policy development;
• provide *services*, such as case management and enabling services, to managed care clients; and
• assist managed care organizations with *assurance and oversight* when working with state agencies with regulatory responsibility.

In carrying out the assessment function, governmental public health agencies have a responsibility to monitor the health status of managed care enrollees, just as for others in their communities. Similarly, governmental agencies must ensure that members of managed care plans have access to quality health care, and assessment results provide relevant information to carry out this function. In conjunction with managed care, these two functions are clearly interrelated and have undeniable costs. Managed care organizations can and should participate in data preparation and analysis, and their data systems can facilitate these activities. If there are to be independent checks on managed care plans' performance, these functions must, at some level, involve public health or other governmental agencies.

BOX 5. Minnesota Department of Health

Minnesota has a relatively mature managed care market and has been licensing health maintenance organizations (HMOs) since the early 1970s. Most of the employer-insured population is enrolled in an HMO, except in rural areas. In 1994, approximately 80% of the Twin Cities population of 2.6 million was enrolled in HMOs, Preferred Provider Organizations, and self-funded employer plans. The State of Minnesota is a large employer that began coordinating health services for its employees in 1989 and joined the Buyers' Health Care Action Group (BHCAG) in 1995. BHCAG is a coalition of 23 area employers that developed a plan to provide direct contracting with competing health systems to develop health care systems that offer a full continuum of services; shared financial risk with purchasers; clinical and fiscal accountability; competition on the basis of quality, cost, and service; and commitment to community-wide quality improvement.

In addition, Minnesota is in the process of transferring its Medicaid enrollees and Aid to Families with Dependent Children recipients into HMOs. It plans—in the event that Congress enacts legislation that creates a block grant system for Medicaid—to take a portion of Medicaid funds and set it aside for the public health infrastructure.

Minnesota requires all HMOs to file annual action and collaboration plans. Action plans provide information to consumers, purchasers, and the community, as a first step toward greater accountability of health plan companies. This is intended to encourage local discussions of the health needs of the community. The Minnesota Department of Health is responsible for ensuring that the action plans submitted by managed care organizations are available for review by local organizations. Collaboration plans describe the actions that managed care organizations intend to take to achieve public health goals for their service areas. Action plan are to be jointly developed in collaboration with community health boards, regional coordinating boards, and other community organizations providing health services within the service area of the managed care organization. Managed care organizations are required to cover services out of network in the area of STDs, AIDS, tuberculosis, and family planning.

Minnesota has a Community Health Services Act that provides the framework for state and local partnerships in that the state delegates most core public health functions to the local level. Community health boards submit a plan every year based upon the community's assessment of its needs. Funds are provided from the state to the community, based upon its needs assessment. Federal preventive health block grants are used to hold capacity-building conferences in specific areas such as immunization, STDs, alcohol and tobacco use, prenatal care, and violence. These conferences bring together representatives from local public health agencies, community health providers, managed care organizations, and other health service providers to analyze the community's needs assessment data.

SOURCES: Based on a presentation by Anne Barry, commissioner of health of Minnesota, at the February 22, 1996 meeting of the Public Health Committee; National Health Policy Forum, 1995; Minnesota Department of Health, 1995a,b.

Roles for Managed Care Organizations

Managed care organizations can also take a more active role in improving the public's health. They can strengthen their health promotion and disease prevention activities by integrating public health programs and services with their primary health care activities and collaborating with public health agencies. With public health agencies and others, managed care organizations can advocate for measures to improve the public's health in the community. Managed care organizations can also develop their data systems to be useful for surveillance and epidemiologic research. Furthermore, they can continue to pave the way for improving the quality of health care (Box 6).

Showstack and colleagues (1996) have argued that managed care organizations have a social responsibility to "broaden their missions from the care of enrolled populations to include contributions to the health of the communities in which they serve." To guide managed care organizations and judge whether they are responsible, accountable, and responsive contributors to the community's health, Showstack and colleagues offer the following eight attributes of a socially responsible managed care system:

1. enrolls a representative segment of the general population living in the system's geographic service area;
2. identifies and acts on opportunities for community health improvement;
3. participates in community-wide data networking and sharing;
4. publishes information regarding its financial performance and contributions to its community;
5. includes the community, broadly defined, in the governance and advisory structures of the managed care system;
6. participates actively in health professions education programs;
7. collaborates meaningfully with academic health centers, health departments, and other components of the public health infrastructure; and
8. advocates publicly for community health promotion and disease prevention policies.

Local health departments can organize as managed care providers and compete with private care plans for payer contracts or they can contract with managed care plans to provide specific services. Public health agencies can also assert their assurance function. They can play a strong regulatory role by setting standards, through licensing, and by monitoring the quality of services (Box 7). These roles, while important, will take time, skill, and initiative to develop. Furthermore, some challenges will arise. For example, there is a potential conflict of interest if public health departments have managed care contracts and are also

BOX 6. U.S. Healthcare

U.S. Healthcare is a large, for-profit company that operates in the northeastern, middle Atlantic, and southeastern United States. It was founded 22 years ago in Pennsylvania and uses an independent physician association model, which means that each physician has a private practice and agrees by contract to accept U.S. Healthcare members. U.S. Healthcare has approximately 2.5 million members, of which 130,000 are Medicare members, 87,000 are Medicaid members, and 10,000 are covered under an uninsured children's program. Each year about 26% of the Medicaid population disenrolls. Only 3.6% of the Medicare population disenrolls, which makes it the most stable group.

U.S. Healthcare's responsibility for public health cuts across many of its programs. These programs include women's health, domestic violence, primary care, and a program that incorporates nutritional screening and interventions into medical practice. Health educators at U.S. Healthcare developed office-based programs to assist physicians working with patients who are enrolled in programs such as smoking cessation. For patient outreach, there are preventive care and immunization programs. Other public health programs include (1) Challenge 1996 to immunize the Medicare population against pneumococcal pneumonia; (2) cancer screening; (3) Medicaid's Early and Periodic Screening, Diagnosis, and Treatment; (4) an uninsured children's program; and (5) health education programs such as *Healthy Breathing* for smoking cessation, *Healthy Lifestyles* to decrease stress, *Healthy Eating* to assist in establishing healthy eating patterns, as well as avoiding obesity, and a fitness program. Case management is also a part of their health care plan. Teams of nurse case managers and social work case managers are formed depending upon the patient population.

Health plan accountability is a major issue for the company, because its management believes it is important to make available performance measurement information that assesses the health plan's effectiveness in providing services and to identify areas for improvement. U.S. Healthcare has been involved in developing the Heath Plan Employer Data and Information Set (HEDIS) and has a representative serving on the Medicaid HEDIS committee and the Medicare HEDIS subcommittee. The Medicare Quality report card was developed by U.S. Healthcare in collaboration with its division, U.S. Quality Algorithms, because the Medicare HEDIS was still being developed at the time and there were no measurements that they could use for their Medicare beneficiary patient population.

SOURCE: Based on a presentation by Sandy Harmon-Weiss, senior vice president and medical director, U.S. Healthcare, at the February 22, 1996, meeting of the Public Health Committee.

BOX 7. San Diego and Los Angeles Counties' Experience with Public Health and Managed Care

SAN DIEGO COUNTY DEPARTMENT OF HEALTH SERVICES

The San Diego County Health Department established a Medi-Cal (California's Medicaid program) managed care system that integrates public health functions and services of a local health department with private-sector health plans. The Medi-Cal managed care contract stipulates that health plans will provide services to the Medicaid population and that the health department will administer the Medi-Cal program. The San Diego County Health Department will be responsible for oversight and enrollment of the program. The State Health Department will be responsible for setting local standards and requirements in the Medi-Cal managed care contracts with managed care organizations.

The San Diego County Health Department will certify physicians who provide public health services for selected communicable diseases and early intervention for children and pregnant women. It will also determine eligibility, will inform patients of their rights and responsibilities in using health care resources, and will enroll people into health plans. The County Health Department will also select performance standards and provide oversight for quality improvement. Local monitoring of health indicators calculated from reports on all health care encounters will be performed for the Medi-Cal population. The County Health Department is also involved with providing public health services (immunizations, home visitation, and teaching responsible parenting) to a new child abuse center (administered by the Social Services Agency).

The County Health Department has created partnerships with representatives of San Diego community organizations (e.g., the San Diego Chamber of Commerce, the San Diego Taxpayers Association, the Medical Society, the Hospital Council, the Welfare Rights Organization, and the Legal Aid Society). Representatives of these organizations meet with the health department staff about public health policies and programs for the community. In this way, the community is involved in the planning process of all new public health programs.

LOS ANGELES COUNTY DEPARTMENT OF HEALTH SERVICES

The Los Angeles County Department of Health Services is also in the process of implementing California's Medi-Cal managed care program. The department developed a memoranda of understanding (MOU) between the Public Health Programs and Services (PHPS) and the Personal Health Services (PHS) branches of the department regarding provision of clinical preventive services and other services provided by PHS that have or could have public health significance. The department also developed MOUs as a basis of negotiation between PHPS and the health maintenance organizations in Los Angeles County intending to participate in the state's Medi-Cal managed care program. The

Continued

> **BOX 7.** *Continued*
>
> MOUs cover both administrative issues and program areas detailing specific tasks and responsibilities. The program areas included in the MOUs are family planning services, sexually transmitted diseases, HIV counseling and testing services, immunizations, children with special health care needs, prenatal care, child health and disability prevention programs, and tuberculosis.
>
> SOURCES: Based on a presentation by Paul Simms, deputy director, Department of Health Services, San Diego County, at the February 22, 1996, meeting of the Public Health Committee; and on a presentation by James Haughton, senior health services policy advisor, County of Los Angeles Department of Health Services, at the October 27, 1995. meeting of the Public Health Committee.

playing a regulatory role with managed care organizations. Despite these challenges, many state and local public health departments have moved forward to develop their abilities in the managed care marketplace.

CONCLUSIONS

There has been substantial growth in organized health care delivery systems (which include managed care organizations) in recent years, and these developments have important implications for the health of the public. In the discussions initiated by the Committee on Public Health, proponents of managed care have argued that its goals and tools are consistent with public health. Many public health professionals, on the other hand, have also indicated concerns about managed care organizations' motives and ability to deliver on their promises. The committee's view, as developed in this section, is that if the proper kinds of partnerships between managed care organizations and governmental public health departments are developed, managed care can indeed make an important contribution to improving the health of the public.

The proliferation of organized health care delivery systems, which continue to provide care for an increasing number of Americans, has made it possible in some locales for governmental public health agencies to assure the provision of personal health services entirely within the private sector. How many elements of public health services private organizations can or should subsume remains unclear, but they can be considerable. Providing care for the uninsured, however, remains a challenge; governmental public health departments will be ill prepared and inadequately funded to do so if no other personal services are being provided.

To ensure that partnerships between governmental public health agencies and managed care organizations work effectively toward improving the health of the public, the committee reiterates *The Future of Public Health* recommendation that **the function of local public health agencies should include "assurance that high-quality services, including personal health services, needed for the protection of public health in the community are available and accessible to all persons. . . ."** This assurance function can be carried out "by encouraging other entities (private or public sector), by requiring such actions through regulation, or by providing services directly." Public health agencies can only exercise this responsibility if they are adequately staffed, equipped, and funded for this complex and demanding task and have appropriate relationships with health service providers. These activities should not be undertaken at the expense of existing essential public health services. Particular concerns arise when health departments have a dual role: direct provision of personal health services to some people and regulating private entities providing similar services to others. To improve the efficiency of all health systems, **health agencies and organized health delivery systems, in conjunction with other community stakeholders, must reach agreement on their proper roles and responsibilities, which will vary by locale.** Successful models of the integration of public health and managed care and of joint approaches to policy development do exist and need to be studied and tested more broadly.

Most public health agencies do not currently have the full statutory and regulatory authority to ensure the accountability of the organized health delivery systems to the public. In the current regulatory structure, health care delivery systems are often regulated by insurance commissions that focus on fiscal integrity rather than health. State Medicaid agencies, usually separate from public health departments, also typically focus on fiscal rather than medical accountability dimensions. Recognizing the clear need for financial oversight, **governmental public health agencies should increase their ability to oversee health care providers, with the goal of becoming coequal partners with insurance regulators and state Medicaid agencies, to ensure that the public's health is addressed in the regulation of public and private health care delivery systems** (see Box 8). In many states, additional legislative authority will be needed before public health agencies can take on this role. This approach requires population-based health outcome and performance standards that can be monitored, and public health agencies should participate in the development and monitoring of these standards.

The functions described in this report cannot be undertaken without properly trained professionals available to all communities. Thus, **public health professionals and students enrolled in schools of public health should be trained to work with health services organizations to ensure quality personal** health services in a community, as an essential element in providing for the health of the public. In addition, public health agencies should actively participate with organizations such as state health professions boards, medical schools, accrediting bodies in planning and policy development.

BOX 8. Maryland's Alliance Between the Health Department and the Insurance Commissioner: An Example for Public Health

Health care reform is not a new concept for the State of Maryland. Maryland's "all-payor system" ensures equity among financing mechanism and has not only held down hospital rates to far less than the national average, but has also maintained the high quality of Maryland's privatized hospital delivery system. For more than 20 years, Maryland's rate increases consistently have been less than the national average. In 1993, HB 1359 created a special insurance program for small businesses that presaged the current Kennedy-Kassebaum bill recently signed into law by President Clinton. Furthermore, Maryland's experience with managed care is vast, with penetration rates being third highest in the nation.

With pride in its health care policy formulations, Maryland recognized the importance of creating a working relationship among the critical agencies that affect the statewide system. With statutory relationships defined in the general HMO statute (between the insurance commissioner and the secretary of the Department of Health and Mental Hygiene) early in 1995, a Memorandum of Agreement was signed by the insurance commissioner, the secretary, and the governor-appointed chairmen of the three major commissions responsible for health care regulations (Planning, Hospital Rate Review, and Ambulatory Care Rate and Information System). This memorandum designed a working relationship and led to the development of the **Maryland Health Care Principles** to which each of the organizations subscribe:

• Ensure every Marylander financial and clinical access to health care.
• Provide services at a reasonable cost.
• Maintain the high quality of Maryland's health care system.
• Improve the health status of individuals, families, and communities through an emphasis on prevention and early intervention services.
• Ensure public accountability through use of reporting criteria, such as health status outcomes and financial reports.
• Promote the sharing of public responsibility costs equitably.
• Ensure long-term financial viability.
• Promote equity among purchasers.

In addition, during the 1996 legislative session, the relationship between the insurance commissioner and the health secretary was further strengthened by defininginterdependent roles for oversight of the Managed Care Organizations (MCOs) that will be responsible for providing care under the Medicaid waiver reform program.

Applications prepared by the MCOs will be jointly reviewed. The Department of Health will assist the insurance commissioner in reviewing solvency claims for the new organizations and the commissioner will review the secretary's capitation rates for payment. A mechanism for joint review of complaints has also been established and a separate Memorandum of Understanding was signed in July 1996 to ensure a continuing relationship between the two organizations.

It is precisely because Maryland understands the evolving health care system that this strategic alliance between public health and the insurance administration has been created. The need for common oversight to assure the organizational integrity from both the fiscal and quality of health services delivery perspective is necessary to assure optimal health care services delivery while maintaining the quality of the evolving health care enterprises for Maryland's employers and taxpayers.

SOURCE: Based on information provided by Martin Wasserman, Secretary of the Maryland Department of Health and Mental Hygiene, 1996.

Public Health and the Community

As discussed above, a wide range of entities (governmental, private, and nonprofit organizations) have an effect on and a stake in a community's health (Patrick and Wickizer, 1995). These entities include health care providers, public health agencies, and community organizations explicitly concerned with health. They also include other governmental agencies, community organizations, private industry, and other entities that do not explicitly, or sometimes even consciously, see themselves as having a health-related role; these include, employers, social service and housing agencies, transportation and justice agencies, and faith communities. Many of the relevant entities are based in and focus their attention on the community in question (Box 9). Others, such as state health departments, federal agencies, managed care organizations, and national corporations that have a broader scope than a single community, often play an essential role in determining local health status (IOM, in press).

The discussions of the Committee on Public Health have led to the conclusion that, as communities try to address their health issues in a comprehensive manner, all of the stakeholders will need to sort out their roles and responsibilities and be held accountable for them (IOM, in press). In most communities, there is only limited experience with collaborative or coordinated efforts among these diverse groups. To work together effectively, they will need a common language and an understanding of the multidimensional nature of the determinants of health. They must also find a way to accommodate diversity in values and goals. Governmental public health agencies have traditionally provided specific services to individuals and to the community at large. Local health departments may need to

BOX 9. Public Health at the Local Level

The Committee on Public Health held a workshop on June 27, 1996, at the CDC in Atlanta, Georgia. The first panel session focused on public health functions at the community level. Panel members included the chief executive officer of DeKalb County, the director of the DeKalb County Health Department, the president of the DeKalb County Local Board of Health, a liaison with the state department of health, and members of community-based organizations. Highlights of the discussion are listed below:

Many local health department provide the only source of primary and preventive care for uninsured populations in their communities. It is not clear that managed care organizations will provide primary and preventive care to uninsured people. There remains a substantial role for public health agencies to assure, and if necessary, to provide those preventive services to uninsured people.

Core public health functions are important at the local level and have been incorporated into the legal structure of a number of health departments. Panel members felt that the core functions of public health as defined in *The Future of Public Health* are important as a basis for organizing, understanding, and evaluating the local public health mission.

In light of an increase in the public's general lack of trust in government, panel members felt that it is important for public health agencies to develop more open communication with the public to build their trust. Additionally, it is important for the private sector to work on building institutional trustworthiness because there are many partnerships between the public and private sectors in the area of public health, which will most likely increase over time.

Panel members discussed how local public health agencies were dealing with decreased funding for their activities. Many local public health agencies have to deal with diminished funding, but many are responding to these changes in different ways.

For example, some local public health departments are collaborating with local managed care plans to provide personal health services to the community.

In some local jurisdictions, the process for setting public health priorities is to preserve only those services that are fee-producing. To preserve the non-income producing programs (e.g., smoking prevention), panel members agreed that it is important to establish participatory advisory groups to educate elected officials and community leaders about different public health activities.

Panel members concluded that public health at the local level can be responsive to the needs of the public and effective in providing services to the community.

SOURCE: Panel discussion at the June 27, 1996 Public Health Committee meeting.

transform themselves to become leaders in organizing a community's resources to enhance its health (Baker et al., 1994, NACCHO Blueprint, 1994; APHA, n.d.).

The Future of Public Health identifies the authorities of federal, state, and local public health agencies in the United States, and makes recommendations about governmental structures to carry out the responsibility of public health. Among other conclusions, *The Future of Public Health* supports the American Public Health Association's Model Standards Committee's concept that "every community must be served by a governmental entity charged with . . . responsibility . . . for providing and assuring public health and safety services." The committee's discussions, however, have shown that many communities in the United States currently lack the ability to provide essential public health services. Some communities have nothing comparable to a local department of health, and the variability in capacity and commitment in those that do is quite large. These facts have led CDC Director David Satcher to comment that China has attempted to ensure that every village has access to a village doctor (formerly know as barefoot doctors) whose major role is to provide health education, screening, and other public health interventions at the community level. It is important, Dr. Satcher feels, that every community in the United States has access to a basic public health unit that provides information and interventions needed to optimize its health (D. Satcher, personal communications, 1996).

POLICY DEVELOPMENT IN PUBLIC HEALTH

The *Future of Public Health* defined policy development as "the process by which society makes decisions about problems, chooses goals and the proper means to reach them, handles conflicting views about what should be done, and allocates resources." This definition suggests that partnerships between public health agencies and community-based organizations are essential if policy development is to be successful. *The Future of Public Health,* however, notes that fragmentation is pervasive and persistent in public health. Fragmentation is "the division of responsibility for health care among multiple, separate individuals and agencies, each with a categorical purpose, and the whole lacking a coherent policy, an integrated direction, and coordinated relationships" (Roemer et al., 1975). Many services of public health agencies are funded by the federal government through a myriad of "categorical programs" aimed at specific underserved populations and specific health problems (DHHS, n.d.-a). For example, prenatal and infant care, immunizations, family planning services, and the prevention of STDs and AIDS are funded through separate streams, some going directly to the local level and others passing through the state or another fiscal intermediary. Some have proposed general block grants, with few restrictions on how these federal funds would be used as a solution to this fragmentation, but others are concerned that unpopular but essential public health programs would not get priority at the state or local level (Brown, 1996). Another alternative are the Performance Partnership Grants proposed by the Department of Health and

Human Services (DHHS, n.d.-b), which would have the local flexibility of block grants and performance measures to ensure accountability. Although the committee was not able to give this issue careful attention, these options deserve further consideration.

One of the key considerations in public health is the extent to which public health policymakers accept the essential political nature of public health and develop ways to work with elected officials (Stivers, 1991). Elected officials face many different and sometimes contradictory expectations and demands from the public (Stark, 1995), and therefore, public health agencies must compete for limited attention. For improving the public's health to become a higher priority, its importance must be made clear to elected officials. Recent research at the county level indicates that when local health officials demonstrate various forms of leadership on public health problems, it is possible to achieve improvements in the health care system (Mirando et al., 1994) and develop support for the public health department through the active advocacy of other community organizations.

COLLABORATION WITH THE COMMUNITY

The Future of Public Health acknowledged that public health policy is formulated and implemented by a wide range of participants, including public health professionals, other health professionals, public officials, and the community (see Box 9). Traditionally, public health was seen as the province of the public health department; but increasingly, government agencies are contracting with private community-based providers to carry out service programs (Baker et al., 1994). In substance abuse, HIV/AIDS, childhood disabilities, and many other areas, there are a growing number of sophisticated organizations that are directly providing personal preventive and care services

In recent years, community advisory boards, planning groups, and coalitions have become common in public health. Currently, community participation through an advisory group or coalition is mandated by a wide range of public health programs addressing tobacco control (the COMMIT and ASSIST projects), substance abuse (Office of Substance Abuse program's community partnership grants), HIV/AIDS (Ryan White Care Act), maternal and child health (Healthy Mothers/Healthy Babies, Healthy Start, Immunization, WIC, and Injury Prevention), and women's health (Breast and Cervical Cancer Screening) (Sofaer, 1992). Community-based organizations of this sort act as "advisors" and "partners" to governmental public health agencies. This latter role involves a long-term mutual commitment, a genuine desire of each partner to understand the other, benefits to each partner that outweigh the costs of the partnership, and meaningful collaboration in defining agendas and action strategies. Through this kind of genuine partnership trust can be established, and this ultimately gets translated into a more powerful system to address community health problems and to advocate for policy support.

Beginning in 1992, the W. K. Kellogg Foundation funded seven community-based public health (CBPH) projects (in California, Georgia, Maryland, Massachusetts, Michigan, North Carolina, and Washington) to link public health agencies and their communities with academic leaders in public health. The primary purpose of this four-year initiative was to implement the recommendations of *The Future of Public Health* to reform professional education by linking it more effectively with practitioners. Kellogg achieved this by connecting both the academic and practice partners with communities that have serious public health problems. Not only were the educational objectives realized, but the initiative enhanced the capacity of all partners to improve the public's health. For the partners, it provided access to new opportunities such as leadership, education, and employment; skills in mobilizing resources; and, of primary importance, an enhanced delivery of services. More specifically, it proved a highly effective way of realizing the potential of public health's core functions. One of the key lessons learned was that genuine partnership with and by members of the community significantly enhances public health education, research, and service—including that which occurs in the practice agencies. The Flint, Michigan project is profiled in Box 10.

When grass-roots communities recognize that public health agencies are their assurance that the health system operates to protect and improve their collective health, they will advocate for the fiscal and regulatory tools to enable the agencies to carry out that role. Rather than being seen as a component of government that taxes them and does things to them, public health agencies can be recognized as the visible expression of the community's desire to collectively address its common health problems. Thus the strategy of forming deep, long-lasting community partnerships is part of the same strategy that can ultimately provide public health agencies with the tools to assure that the managed care system operates to the benefit of the health of the public as awhole.

DIFFICULT PROBLEMS AND DIFFICULTY SOLVING PROBLEMS

In a democratic and pluralistic society, such as in the United States, public policy-making in practice is not a rational or neutral process. Instead, it is a dynamic and political process that involves a constant struggle of ideas and interests (Stone, 1988). Sometimes this process is disjointed and incremental;

BOX 10. Community-Based Public Health: Genesee County, Michigan

The Flint and Vicinity Action Community and Economic Development Corporation (FACED) is a member of a partnership in Genesee County, Michigan, comprising community members, community-based neighborhood organizations, the University of Michigan, and the Genesee County Health Department. Along with organizational counterparts in the City of Detroit, this Michigan consortium is one of seven state partnerships funded by the W.K. Kellogg Foundation to improve the public's health through the practice of community-based public health (CBPH).

FACED was begun by a group of ministers who were confronted regularly in their congregations with a broad range of economic, social and health dilemmas. CBPH facilitated the formation of a nonprofit organization through which their ministry could be expressed. CBPH subsequently contributed to the organization's financial, business, administrative, and technical capacities. Among current activities, FACED now transports community residents for health care appointments, coordinates the work of seven "church health teams," orients local residents to services offered through community agencies, trains and develops other organizations, and delivers tobacco use prevention programming.

Over the four years of the CBPH partnership, wide gaps in culture, race, trust, orientation, and history have been bridged among team members whose experience working jointly now forms the foundation for work with an expanded network of community residents and organizations. Experiences helping to pass local tobacco control regulations, successful advocacy in the area of lead poisoning prevention and abatement, and work along with other partners to begin fact-finding in association with a potential case of environmental discrimination were also described.

The active and supportive presence of the CBPH partnership enabled organizations to: both preserve and lose their traditional identity dependent upon the special challenges of the task; recognize and value the "voice" of community residents; and be adaptive in the design and funding of programming and research.

SOURCE: Based on a presentation by Yvonne Lewis, program coordinator of the Flint and Vicinity Action Community Economic Development, Inc., at the June 27, 1996, meeting of the Public Health Committee.

---

other times it is more erratic and random (Lindblom, 1959; Kingdon, 1995). Public health, like other areas of public policy such as education or criminal justice, faces internal and external struggles in the development and implementation of policy. These challenges include conflicting and competing values and goals, struggles with defining and resolving problems, and obstacles to the implementation of programs. Additionally, in recent years, a growing public mistrust of government, government institutions, and politics has created other challenges to society (Box 11).

BOX 11. Public Trust and Confidence in Government

Americans have had conflicting attitudes about government since the founding of this country. There is strong individualism in the United States that often leads to suspicion of government and the restraints that may be placed on the individual. However, the public does recognize the role that government can play in helping individuals and organizations achieve certain goals. In recent years, there has been a growing mistrust of government, government institutions, and politics in general. The public often has higher expectations of government agencies than of private-sector organizations and expects public officials to be scrupulously honest, to avoid conflicts of interest, to perform their jobs efficiently, and to be publicly accountable. The misdeeds of government officials are often printed on the front pages of newspapers. In addition, the number of large, technically oriented public agencies and private industries have increased, while at the same time public support for large-scale scientific and technological developments has decreased. However, there are some things that governmental agencies can do to build public trust and confidence.

Trust is the belief that those with whom one interacts will take one's interests into account, even in situations in which one is not in a position to recognize, evaluate, or thwart a potentially negative course of action by those trusted. **Confidence** exists when the party trusted is believed to be able to empathize with one's interests, is competent to act on that empathy, and will go to considerable lengths to keep her or his word. **Trustworthiness** is a combination of trust and confidence.

An erosion of public trust in governmental agencies will take hold when the following perceptions and beliefs become widespread.

Benefits and Costs:

• There is a perceived mismatch in the distribution of benefits and the costs associated with realizing the agency's mission.

• The risk of hazard from program failure is perceived to be very high and very long lasting.

Accuracy and Speed of Feedback:

• High levels of technical, esoteric knowledge are required to conduct the agency's mission or to evaluate its success, risk, and hazards.

• A long lag occurs in the time to the discovery of success or failure, especially if the evidence of failure is likely to be ambiguous and equivocal.

Capability of Others to Meet Expectations:

• There is a perceived decline in the competence of agency members relative to the demands posed by the problems central to effective operations.

• There is a perceived decline in operating reliability and in complete disclosure of information about difficulties and failures.

Continued

BOX 11. *Continued*

Motivation of Others to Understand and Keep Bargains:
- There is a perceived unwillingness to respect the views of the vulnerable parties.
- There is a perceived inability to fulfill promises to maintain consistent levels of agency performance or promised public political support.

There are several things that a governmental agency can do to establish and maintain public trust and confidence within its organization and external to its organization. Increasing institutional trustworthiness begins with its internal operations. An agency should commit itself and its contractors to maintain a high level of professional and managerial competence. It should establish and meet reasonable technical performance measures and schedule milestones that are dictated by a project's scientific requirements and pursue technical options and strategies that can be clearly demonstrated to broad segments of the public. It should reward honest self-assessment that permits the organization to solve problems that have been identified internally before they are discovered by outsiders. In addition, the agency should move the responsibility for promoting and protecting the internal efforts to sustain public trust and confidence throughout the organization.

For an agency to build trust and confidence with the public, it should establish an advisory board at the state and local levels as well as at the national level that includes all interested parties in the work of the agency. The agency's top-level staff should be accessible to citizens and their representatives. Open communication with the community and agency constituents is crucial to developing institutional trustworthiness. It is important to establish consistent and respectful efforts to reach out to state and community leaders and the general public for the purpose of informing, consulting, and collaborating with them about the technical and operational aspects of the agency's work and activities.

SOURCES: Based on a presentation by Todd LaPorte, professor of political sciences, University of California at Berkeley, at the June 27, 1996 meeting of the Public Health Committee; LaPorte, 1994; Feingold, 1995; and LaPorte and Metlay, in press.

Many problems such as violence, substance abuse, and teen pregnancy are fundamentally difficult because they have multiple, intertwined medical, social, and economic causes (Sommer, 1995; Yates, 1977). Resolving these problems requires a comprehensive, collaborative response from different public agencies and private organizations, including but not limited to public health. For example, addressing the problem of lead poisoning prevention involves a coordinated strategy among governmental public health agencies, the medical community, environmental, occupational health, and housing agencies, business, labor, and the general public as well as the public education system.

For other problems, the solutions seem more straightforward, yet the scientific evidence about the efficacy and cost-effectiveness of solutions has been elusive (Council on Linkages, 1995). Policymakers need to know what types of interventions are available, which ones have been shown to be effective, how much they cost, and whether they can be modified and adapted to local circumstances (Holtgrave et al., 1996). Practitioners in governmental public health agencies need the confidence and funding to sustain new models of practice while maintaining models proven to be successful. The federal government has begun to document the effectiveness of public health interventions (DHHS, N.d.-b; Gordon et al., 1996), and this research has begun to be translated into practice. For example, evidence has accumulated that use of mammography can reduce the mortality due to breast cancer among women 50 years and older by 30%, and the Pap test has been shown to be an effective technology for reducing cervical cancer mortality (Henson et al., 1996). In 1990, with passage of the Breast and Cervical Cancer Mortality Prevention Act, the Centers for Disease Control and Prevention (CDC) established a comprehensive public health program to increase access to breast and cervical cancer screening services for women who are medically underserved. This program has dramatically increased the number of older women screened for breast and cervical cancer (Henson et al., 1996). Additional efforts are underway through CDC to improve the database on effective community-based interventions (CDC, 1996).

Even when promising solutions exist, public health agencies too often have difficulty generating support for interventions among elected officials and the general public. Programs to improve the public's health compete with medical care services for attention and resources. While medical care services treat urgent problems, many public health programs prevent problems from occurring or progressing. Thus the benefits of medical care are often more tangible and concrete, while the benefits of public health are more diffuse and less well appreciated.

A key struggle for governmental public health leaders and those in the private and nonprofit sectors with an economic, ethical, or philosophical interest in the public's health is making the benefits of community-based, population-wide public health activities and initiatives more recognizable, and finding allies who will speak on behalf of these initiatives and the unique role for governmental public health agencies in carrying out these initiatives. A good example of this is the way that advocates at the state and local levels have been able to demonstrate how the general public is affected by the costs of smoking: paying the medical costs of lung cancer patients through higher insurance premiums or taxes for public programs, experiencing the effects of passive smoking, and the numerous allies in the communities who have embraced the tobacco-free movement. In contrast, public health policymakers have been somewhat less successful in generating support or alliances for HIV/AIDS prevention or STD control in part because of the incorrect perceptions that these are not widespread problems in the general population, that STDs do not have severe consequences, and because of the public's reluctance to be open about sexuality (IOM, 1996). Public health agencies need to work with the community to identify common problems that both can work on together.

Some have suggested that public health agencies be compared to police and fire departments in a public safety context (Box 12). Others suggest that because the unique role of public health agencies relates directly to prevention and the community, it would be helpful to emphasize health protection, disease prevention, and health promotion (Baker et al., 1994). Emphasizing the Public Health Functions Steering Committee's vision statement for governmental public health agencies—"Healthy People in Healthy Communities"—might be a fruitful approach.

BOX 12. A Metaphor for Public Health

Public health agencies are a lot like fire departments. They teach and practice prevention at the same time that they maintain readiness to take on emergencies. They are most appreciated when they respond to emergencies. They are most successful—and least noticed—when their prevention measures work the best.

In another respect, the two are different. Everyone knows what a fire department does; few know what a public health department does. The very existence of health departments is testament to the fact that, when legislators, county commissioners, and other policymakers understand what those departments do, they support them. It is a rare person who, once familiar with the day-to-day activities of a public health department, would want to live in a community without a good one.

SOURCE: Washington State Department of Health, 1994.

CONCLUSIONS

In its discussions with community group representatives and public health officials, the committee heard of many innovative and effective approaches to community partnerships and collaboration that are consistent with widespread themes regarding community development and "reinventing government." Broader application and further development of these new approaches to collaboration within government (with legislators, boards of health, and nonhealth agencies) and with community partners to achieve public health goals should be encouraged.

Shared responsibility, however, requires careful management. **The governmental public health agency in each community needs to be capable of identifying and working with all of the entities that influence a community's** health, especially those that are not directly health related. This function must be undertaken by public health agencies that understand the interactions of the full range of factors that influence the community's health. To address this, a companion IOM report proposes a "community health improvement process" that draws on performance monitoring concepts, an understanding of community development, and the role of public health consistent with the Committee on Public Health's discussions (IOM, in press). Public health professionals who must work with a community to improve its own health need to be trained and their roles need to be upgraded or enhanced.

The committee's discussions showed that many functions essential to the public's health, such as immunizations and health education, can be and are now being performed by either public or private entities, depending on the historical context, community resources, and political dynamics of a particular area. Some functions, however, such as environmental regulation and enforcement of public health laws, must remain the responsibility of governmental public health agencies. There also needs to be a resource in each community to ensure that the health impact of multiple interventions in the community are understood and addressed. This remains an ideal function for governmental public health agencies and should not be delegated. Thus, the committee reasserts the critical findings of *The Future of Public Health* that governmental public health agencies have a unique function in the community: "to see to it that vital elements are in place and that the [public health] mission is adequately addressed." These elements include assessment, policy development, and assurance. For a governmental agency to execute this responsibility effectively, there must be explicit legal authority as well as health goals and functions, that the public understands and demands. A fundamental building block for this new approach to governance is public trust. With trust in public institutions at risk or at low levels in many communities, governmental public health agencies must find ways to improve communication and openness with the public to maintain and increase their trustworthiness.

Revisiting *The Future of Public Health*

In the course of its discussions about current public health issues, the Committee on Public Health had the opportunity to readdress the findings and conclusions of *The Future of Public Health*, and to assess the impact that the report has had on the field. If not begun directly in response to *The Future of Public Health*, then many of the following activities were at least informed and energized by it.

BETTER DEFINITIONS OF PUBLIC HEALTH

One of the most valuable aspects of *The Future of Public Health* was the articulation of the mission and functions of governmental public health agencies (see Introduction). Specifying the functions of public health enabled federal, state, and local health departments to begin a dialogue and assessment about what they do and whether it was appropriate and adequate. This clarification of the roles for public health agencies was part of a larger movement to reinvent and reorganize governmental public health programs to make them more efficient and effective and to build support from public officials and the general public (University of Illinois, 1994).

From the core functions identified in *The Future of Public Health*, experts developed more specific frameworks of public health processes. Miller and colleagues developed 10 public health practices, each linked to one of the core functions (Miller, 1995; see also Box 13). This framework was then used to assess the performance of local health departments (Miller et al., 1994).

BOX 13. Public Health Practices

ASSESSMENT PRACTICES

(The regular systematic collection, assembly, analysis, and dissemination of information on the health of the community.)

1. Asses the health needs of the community by establishing a systematic needs assessment process that periodically provides information the health status and health needs of the community.

2. Investigate the occurrence of adverse health effects and health hazards in the community by conducting timely investigations that identify the magnitude of health problems including their duration, trends, location, and populations at risk.

3. Analyze the determinants of identified health needs to identify etiologic and contributing factors that place certain segments of the population at risk for adverse health outcomes.

POLICY DEVELOPMENT PRACTICES

(The exercise of the responsibility to serve the public interest in the development of comprehensive public health policies by promoting the use of the scientific knowledge base in decision making.)

4. Advocate for public health, build constituencies and identify resources in the community by generating supportive and collaborative relationships with public and private agencies and constituent groups for the effective planning, implementation and management of public health activities.

5. Set priorities among health needs based on the size and seriousness of the problems, the acceptability, economic feasibility and effectiveness of interventions.

6. Develop plans and policies to address priority health needs by establishing goals and objectives to be achieved through a systematic course of action that focuses on local community needs and equitable distribution of resources and involves the participation of constituents and other related governmental agencies.

ASSURANCE PRACTICES

(The assurance to constituents that services necessary to achieve agreed-on goals are provided by encouraging actions of others (private or public), requiring action through regulation, or providing service directly.)

7. Manage resources; develop organizational structure through the acquisition, allocation, and control of human, physical, and fiscal resources; and maximize the operation functions of the local public health system through coordination of community agencies' efforts and avoidance of duplication of services.

8. Implement programs and other arrangements ensuring or providing direct services for priority health needs identified in the community by taking actions that translate plans and policies into services.

9. Evaluate programs, provide quality assurance in accordance with applicable professional and regulatory standards to ensure that programs are consistent with plans and policies, and provide feedback on inadequacies and changes needed to redirect programs and resources.

10. Inform and educate the public on public health issues of concern in the community, promote an awareness about public health services' availability, and health education initiatives that contribute to individual and collective changes in health knowledge, attitudes, and practices achieve a healthier community.

SOURCES: Miller et al., 1994; Turnock and Handler, 1995

The National Association for County and City Health Officials, working from the goal of healthy people in healthy communities, developed a paradigm for a community's health system. The paradigm incorporates ten elements, each of which must be present for a health system in a community to be considered complete (NACHO and CDC, 1994). In this framework, the role of the governmental public health agency is to assess whether the elements are present— either on its own or in partnership with others; to develop legal or financial incentives for the ten elements; or through its own efforts to provide the ten elements or a subset of the elements, based on local priority setting, if others cannot be found to provide, will not provide, or are unable to provide elements of a high quality to meet community benchmarks.

The maternal and child health (MCH) community also expanded upon the list of ten essential services to develop an MCH Functions Framework (Grason and Guyer, 1995). This framework details MCH program functions and provides examples of local, state, and federal activities for implementing MCH program functions. It has been used as a strategic planning, evaluation, and educational tool by state and local MCH programs and schools.

While *The Future of Public Health* has had an important impact on public health professionals, health officials have not yet found the correct formula for informing the public about the importance of public health. Finding better ways to inform the public and elected officials of the substance and importance of public health clearly deserves more attention.

PUBLIC HEALTH CAPACITY

By clarifying goals within the profession and supplying tools for advocacy, *The Future of Public Health* provided a stimulus for activities to strengthen the capacity of public health. Although there is still tremendous variability in capacity among state and local public health agencies, over the past eight years, there have been many targeted areas in which public health capacity has improved. Two important areas have been in response to the resurgence of tuberculosis and the increase in childhood vaccine-preventable disease, both occurring in the late 1980s and early 1990s. A heavy infusion of federal funds and a reorganized operationally focused tuberculosis program enabled New York City to reverse the increase in cases (Frieden et al., 1995). In response to outbreaks of measles, mumps, and other childhood diseases, the federal government dramatically increased appropriations for immunization, and immunization action planning projects were initiated in cities and states across the country (Woods and Mason, 1992). Another important area has been in small rural communities. Some local health departments find that *The Future of Public Health* report is valuable in helping to direct public health activities (Box 14).

At the state level, *The Future of Public Health* spawned a series of activities intended to clarify and strengthen the core functions of public health. These include the State of Washington's Public Health Improvement Plan (Washington State Department of Health, 1994) and the Illinois public health improvement plan (Illinois Department of Public Health, 1990, 1993, and 1994).

Currently, 69% of the expenditures of state and local health departments are used to provide personal health care services (Eilbert et al., 1996). Funding for these personal services from federal and state sources such as Medicaid help pay for administrative and other functions. Thus, as revenue streams for services to vulnerable populations shift from public health departments to managed care organizations, the financial base for governmental public health agencies could shrink. In light of new roles for public health agencies to work with managed care organizations and the community as outlined above, some states have begun to explore ways to reinvest in local public health agencies (Re-Investment Work Group, 1995). This will require public health officials and their allies to inform state legislatures about what public health agencies do in the state and community and their contributions to the public's health.

PRACTICE GUIDELINES FOR PREVENTION

It became clear to public health professionals that to improve the public's health further, it was necessary to develop guidelines for practice and prevention.

BOX 14. Barron County Health Department, Wisconsin

Barron County is a rural community in Wisconsin that is distant from any metropolitan area. Because it is difficult to get current public health information, Barron County has relied on *The Future of Public Health*. The report has provided valuable information that the County Health Department has used in managing the community's public health activities.

Some recent activities in Wisconsin and Barron County demonstrate the relevance of *The Future of Public Health*. The State of Wisconsin has used many of the report's recommendations. It has published its own version of *Healthier People in Wisconsin: An Agenda for the Year 2000*. It recently revised *Wisconsin Public Health Statutes 1993* to define a health planning and leadership role for local health departments that is fundamental to the protection of the health of the community. The three core functions of a local health department identified in the statutes are assessment, policy development, and assurance.

In 1995, these documents provided the Barron County Health Department the impetus to assume the lead in a countywide process to assess the health of Barron County using the National Association for County and City Health Officials' APEXPH (Assessment Protocol for Excellence in Public Health). The goal was to assess the county's health needs, develop policies to meet those needs, and to ensure that quality services (including personal health services) that are necessary for the protection of public health are available and accessible to all persons in Barron County.

The APEXPH process has been successful. The community has renewed confidence in the Barron County Board of Health. Since the completion of the Barron County Health Plan 2000 in December 1995, the Board has passed two county ordinances to protect the public's health, and it continues to involve the community by requesting input from other government agencies and community organizations on health concerns, department programs, and fiscal matters.

SOURCE: Based on information provided by Kathy Newman, director of the Barron County Health Department, 1996; NACCHO, 1991.

The Council on Linkages, with support from the W. K. Kellogg Foundation, sponsored a "Guideline Development Project for Public Health Practice." The goals of this project were to assess the desirability and feasibility of practice guidelines and to test a methodology for evaluating the scientific evidence on which such guidelines could be built. Four public health problems were chosen for study: (1) immunization of children, (2) treatment for tuberculosis, (3) prevention of cardiovascular disease, and (4) prevention of lead poisoning. This project found that the development of public health practice guidelines is feasible and should be pursued (Council on Linkages, 1995), and efforts are underway to develop prototype guidelines.

The CDC has also begun to assess the effectiveness of community-based prevention guidelines. They have collected these guidelines into a "Prevention Guidelines Database," available to practitioners though CDC's PC Wonder (Friede et al., 1993), an on-line electronic communication system, and the Internet (Gordon et al., 1996). The CDC is providing staff support to a newly established U.S. Task Force on Community Preventive Services intended to complement the U.S. Preventive Services Task Force *Guide to Clinical Preventive Services* (DHHS, 1989, 1996), which is designed for practitioners to use with individual patients. The proposed new guide will focus on community-based prevention and control strategies.

TRAINING OF PUBLIC HEALTH PROFESSIONALS

The Future of Public Health identified needs and gaps in the training of public health professionals, which were further addressed at an IOM Conference on Education, Training, and the Future of Public Health held in 1987 (IOM, 1991). *The Future of Public Health* called for strengthening the links between schools of public health and public health agencies. In 1988, the Health Resources and Services Administration and the CDC established a "Public Health Faculty/ Agency Forum" to develop universal and discipline-specific competencies and recommendations (Sorensen and Bialek, 1991). These competencies are now being used by public health schools and programs to guide the development of curriculums and by agencies to assess needs for training.

The forum's work led to formation of the "Council on Linkages Between Academia and Public Health Practice." The council is working to improve practice in public health agencies and education by refining and implementing the recommendations of the Public Health Faculty/Agency Forum, establishing links between academia and the agencies of the public health community, and creating a process for continuing public health education throughout one's career (Sorensen and Bialek, 1991).

DEVELOPING STRONGER LEADERS AND PRACTITIONERS

The Future of Public Health identified serious gaps in the leadership skills of governmental public health leaders and others interested in improving the public's health, including difficulty with the interaction of technical expertise and political accountability, lack of management skills, a high turnover and lack of continuity of leaders, inadequate national leadership, a lack of supportive relationships with the medical community, and insufficient capability in working with the community (IOM, 1988). Roper (1994) notes that public health leaders must understand and deal with multidimensional problems. The straightforward challenges of the past (e.g., developing a vaccine for an uncomplicated infectious disease) have given way to problems such as teen pregnancy, drug abuse, and STDs that are intertwined with seemingly intractable social and economic problems. Even active and experienced public health professionals, Roper reports, are not prepared for current and future challenges and, worse yet, suffer from problems of morale, skills, and systems. These conditions demand that today's leaders in public health be equipped differently than the leaders of yesterday.

Since the IOM's report was released, leadership institutes have been developed at the federal, regional, and state levels. The CDC and the Western Consortium for Public Health established a training institute for state and local public health practitioners at the national level. Regional leadership institutes have been organized at the University of Washington, University of North Carolina, and St. Louis University Schools of Public Health and in the states of Florida, Illinois, Michigan, Missouri, Ohio, and Texas (Gordon et al., 1996).

The CDC has developed an "Information Network for Public Health Officials" (INPHO). This federal-state partnership is designed to connect public health professionals so that they may have access to current data and information to make informed decisions and to provide a vehicle for data exchange. INPHO computer networks and software link organizations eliminate geographic and bureaucratic barriers to communication and information exchange. Georgia was the first state to join the network, and INPHO projects are underway in 13 states. The CDC has also developed a "Public Health Training Network," a distance learning system comprising public, private, and academic partnerships. This network will use computers and satellite systems to train public health professionals and health care providers in the latest issues in public health, such as managed care (Baker et al., 1994; Gordon et al., 1996).

CONCLUSIONS

Through its analysis of the interactions between managed care organizations and the role of governmental public health agencies in enhancing the health of the community and through its discussions about the many responses to *The Future of Public Health*, the committee found that the constructs of the mission and substance of governmental public health agencies envisioned in that report have been extraordinarily useful in revitalizing the infrastructure and rebuilding the federal, state, and local public health system in the United States. These agencies continue to be a fundamental building block in efforts to improve the public's health for the future. However, although clear progress has been made, some of the recommendations of that report have not yet been achieved. In light of this, the committee's analysis shows that **the concepts in** *The Future of Public Health* **remain vital and essential to current and future efforts to energize and focus the efforts of public health. These concepts need to be advanced, applied, and taught to all health professionals.**

The committee also found that **the concepts of assessment, policy development, and assurance**, while useful in the public health community itself, have been difficult to translate into effective messages for key stakeholders, including elected officials and community groups. These concepts **need to be translated into a vernacular that these groups understand.**

In conclusion, the committee found that the public health enterprise in the United States, as embodied in governmental public health agencies, is necessarily diverse in organization and function, but operates within the common framework set out in *The Future of Public Health*. The committee's discussions, however, revealed continuing evidence of inadequate support for governmental public health in many communities. Now, as nearly a decade before, **society must reinvest in governmental public health agencies, with resources, commitments, and contributions from government, private, and nonprofit sectors and substantial legal authorities, if the public's health is to improve.** The partnerships that are the focus of this report—between governmental public health agencies and managed care organizations, and between public health and the community—can provide both political support and a vehicle for this reinvestment.

References

APHA (American Public Health Association). N.d. 95211(PP): *The Role of Public Health in Ensuring Healthy Communities.* Washington, D.C.: APHA.

Atkinson WL, Orenstein WA, and Krugman S. 1992. The Resurgence of Measles in the United States, 1989 and 1990. *Annual Review of Medicine* 43:451–463.

Baker EL, Melton RJ, Stange PV, et al. 1994. Health Reform and the Health of the Public: Forging Community Health Partnerships. *Journal of the American Medical Association* 272(16):1276–1282.

Berwick DM. 1989. Continuous Improvement as an Ideal in Health Care. *New England Journal of Medicine* 320:53–56.

Brown ER. 1996. President's Column. *The Nation's Health.* Washington, D.C.: American Public Health Association.

Brownson RC and Kreuter MW. In press. Future Trends Affecting Public Health: Challenges and Opportunities. *Journal of Public Health Management and Practice.*

CDC (Centers for Disease Control and Prevention). 1996. *Guide to Community Preventive Services.* Atlanta: CDC.

CDC. 1995. *HIV/AIDS Surveillance Report* 7(2).

CDC and GHAA (Group Health Association of America). N.d. *Public Health Agencies and Managed Care: Partnerships for Health.* Atlanta: CDC.

Council on Linkages Between Academia and Public Health Practice. 1995. *Practice Guidelines for Public Health: Assessment of Scientific Evidence, Feasibility, and Benefits.* Albany, N.Y.: Public Health Practice Guidelines Development Project.

51

DHHS (U.S. Department of Health and Human Services). N.d.-a. *For a Healthy Nation: Returns on Investment in Public Health.* Washington, D.C.: DHHS.

DHHS. N.d.-b. *Performance Measurement in Selected Public Health Programs: 1995–1996 Regional Meetings.* Washington, D.C.: Office of the Assistant Secretary for Health, DHHS.

DHHS. 1996. *Guide To Clinical Preventive Services* (Second Edition). A Report of the U.S. Preventive Services Task Force. Washington, D.C.: DHHS.

DHHS. 1991. *Healthy People 2000: National Health Promotion and Disease Prevention Objectives.* Washington, D.C.: DHHS.

DHHS. 1989. *Guide to Clinical Preventive Services. A Report of the U.S. Preventive Services Task Force.* Washington, D.C.: DHHS.

Dionne EJ. 1991. *Why Americans Hate Politics.* New York: Simon & Schuster.

Eilbert KW, Barry MA, Bialek RG, et al. 1996. *Measuring Expenditures for Essential Public Health Services.* Washington, D.C.: Public Health Foundation.

Evans RG, and Stoddart GL. 1994. Producing Health, Consuming Health Care. *Why Are Some People Healthy and Others Not? The Determinants of Health of Populations.* New York: Aldine De Gruyter.

Feingold E. 1995. The Defeat of Health Care Reform: Misplaced Mistrust in Government. *American Journal of Public Health* 85:1619–1622.

Friede A, Taylor WR, and Nadelman L. 1993. On-Line Access to a Cost-Benefit/Cost-Effectiveness Analysis Bibliography via CDC WONDER. *Medical Care* 31(7):JS12–JS17.

Frieden TR, Fujiwara PI, Washko RM, and Hamburg, M. 1995. Tuberculosis in New York City—Turning the Tide. *New England Journal of Medicine* 333:229–233.

Gabel J, Liston D, Jensen G, and Marsteller J. 1994. DataWatch: The Health Insurance Picture in 1993: Some Rare Good News. *Health Affairs* 13(1):327–336.

Gittler J. 1994. Controlling Resurgent Tuberculosis: Public Health Agencies, Public Policy, and the Law. *Journal of Health Politics, Policy, and Law* 19(1):107–147.

Gordon RL, Baker EL, Roper WL, and Omenn GS. 1996. Prevention and the Reforming U.S. Health Care System: Changing Roles and Responsibilities for Public Health. *Annual Review of Public Health* 17:489–509.

Grason H, and Guyer B. 1995. *Public Health Program Functions: Essential Public Health Services to Promote Maternal and Child Health in America.* Baltimore, Md.: Johns Hopkins University Child and Adolescent Health Policy Center.

Green LW, and Kreuter MW. 1990. Health Promotion as a Public Health Strategy for the 1990s. *Annual Review of Public Health* 11:319–334.

Health Resources and Services Administration (HRSA). N.d. Bureau of Primary Health Care's comprehensive managed care program.

Henson RM, Wyatt SW, and Lee NC. 1996. The National Breast and Cervical Cancer Early Detection Program: A Comprehensive Public Health Response to Two Major Health Issues for Women. *Journal of Public Health Practice* 2(2):36–47.

Holtgrave DR, Qualls NL, and Graham JD. 1996. *Annual Review of Public Health* 17:467–488.

Illinois Department of Public Health. 1994. *Project Health: The Reengineering of Public Health in Illinois (A special report issued by the Local Health Liaison Committee).* Springfield, IL.

Illinois Department of Public Health. 1993. *Statewide Health Needs Assessment: Towards a Healthy Illinois 2000.* Springfield, IL.

Illinois Department of Public Health. 1990. *The Road to Better Health: For all of Illinois.* Springfield, IL.

IOM (Institute of Medicine). In press. *Improving Health in the Community: A Role for Performance Monitoring.* Washington, D.C.: National Academy Press.

IOM. 1996. *The Hidden Epidemic: Confronting Sexually Transmitted Diseases.* Washington, D.C.: National Academy Press.

IOM. 1991. *Conference on Education, Training, and the Future of Public Health: Conference Proceedings.* Washington, D.C.: Institute of Medicine.

IOM. 1993. *Access to Health Care in America.* Washington, D.C.: National Academy Press.

IOM. 1988. *The Future of Public Health.* Washington, D.C.: National Academy Press.

Joint Council of Governmental Public Health Agencies. 1996. *Improving the Public's Health: Collaborations Between Public Health Departments and Managed Care Organizations.* Vergennes, Vt.: Wendy Knight & Associates.

Jones C. 1984. *Introduction to the Study of Public Policy.* Monterey, Calif.: Brooks/Cole.

Kaiser Commission on the Future of Medicaid. 1995. *Medicaid and Managed Care: Lessons from the Literature.* Menlo Park, Calif.: Henry J. Kaiser Family Foundation.

Kelley DK, Barnow BS, Gold WA, et al. 1993. *An Analysis of the Federal and State Roles in the Immunization of Preschool Children.* Washington, D.C.: Lewin-VHI.

Kingdon JW. 1995. *Agendas, Alternatives, and Public Policies.* New York: Harper Collins.

LaPorte TR. 1994. Large Technical Systems, Institutional Surprises, and Challenges to Political Legitimacy. *Technology in Society* 16:269–288.

LaPorte TR and Metlay DS. In press. Facing a Deficit of Trust: Hazards and Institutional Trustworthiness. *Public Administration Review*.

Lindblom CE. 1959. The Science of Muddling Through. *Public Administration Review* 19(2):79–88.

Lipson DJ, and Naierman N. 1996. Effects of Health System Changes on Safety Net Providers. *Health Affairs* 15(2):33–48.

McGinnis JM, and Foege WH. 1993. Actual Causes of Death in the United States. *Journal of the American Medical Association* 270(18):2207–2212.

Miller CA. 1995. Letter to the Editor. *American Journal of Public Health* 85(9):1296–1297.

Miller CA, Moore KS, Richards TB, et al. 1994. A Proposed Method for Assessing the Performance of Local Public Health Functions and Practices. *American Journal of Public Health* 84(11):1743–1749.

Minnesota Department of Health. 1995a. 1995 Collaboration Plans. St. Paul.

Minnesota Department of Health. 1995b. Collaboration Between Managed Care Organizations, Local Public Health Systems and the Community. St. Paul.

Mirando VL, Melchior AC, and Sokolow AD. 1994. *Public Health on the Agenda of Counties*. College Park: Department of Government and Politics, The University of Maryland.

National Health Policy Forum. 1995. Site Visit Report (Minneapolis/St. Paul and New Ulm, Minnesota, November 13–15, 1995). Washington, D.C.: George Washington University.

NACHO and CDC (National Association of County Health Officials and the Centers for Disease Control and Prevention). 1994. *Blueprint for a Healthy Community: A Guide for Local Health Departments*. Washington, D.C.: NACHO.

NACHO (National Association of County Health Officials). 1991. *Assessment Protocol for Excellence in Public Health*. Washington, DC: National Association of County and City Health Officials.

NCQA (National Committee for Quality Assurance). 1993. *Health Plan Employer Data and Information Set and User's Manual, Version 2.0* (HEDIS 2.0). Washington, D.C.: NCQA.

Osborne D, and Gaebler T. 1992. *Reinventing Government: How the Entrepreneurial Spirit is Transforming the Public Sector*. Reading, Mass.: Harper Collins.

OTA (Office of Technology Assessment). 1993. *The Continuing Challenge of Tuberculosis* (OTA-H-574). Washington, D.C.: Harper Collins.

Patrick DL, and Wickizer TM. 1995. "Community and Health." In *Society and Health*, B.C. Amick, S Levine, AR Tarlov, and DC Walsh, eds., New York: Oxford University Press.

Re-Investment Work Group. 1995. *Essential Public Health Services: The Case for Reinvestment.* Tampa, Fl.: College of Public Health, University of South Florida.

Reiser, SJ. 1996. Medicine and Public Health: Pursuing a Common Destiny. *Journal of the American Medical Association* 276(17):1429-1430.

Robins LS, and Backstrom C. 1994. The Role of State Health Departments in Formulating Policy: A Survey on the Case of AIDS. *American Journal of Public Health* 84(6):905–909.

Robinson, JC. 1996. Dynamics and Limits of Corporate Growth in Health Care. *Health Affairs* 15(2):155–169.

Roemer R, Kramer C, and Frink JE. 1975. Fragmentation of Health Services. In *Planning Urban Health Services.* New York: Springer.

Roper WL. 1994. Why the Problem of Public Health Leadership? *Leadership in Public Health.* New York: Milbank Memorial Fund.

Rosenbaum S, and Richards TB. 1996. Medicaid Managed Care and Public Health Policy. *Journal of Public Health Management and Practice* 2(3):76–82.

San Diego County Department of Health Services. 1996. Healthy San Diego. San Diego, California.

Showstack J, Lurie N, Leatherman S, et al. 1996. Health of the Public: The Private Sector Challenge. *Journal of the American Medical Association* 276(13)1071-1074.

Sofaer S. 1992. *Coalitions and Public Health: A Program Manager's Guide to the Issues.* Paper prepared for AIDS Communication Support Project, Contract No. 200-91-0906. Washington, D.C.: Academy for Educational Development.

Sommer A. 1995. Wither Public Health? *Public Health Reports* 110:657–661.

Sorensen AA, and Bialek RG, eds. 1991. *The Public Health Faculty/Agency Forum: Linking Graduate Education and Practice, Final Report.* Gainesville: University Press of Florida.

Stark, S. 1995. Too Representative Government. *Atlantic Monthly* 92–106.

Stone DA. 1988. *Policy Paradox and Political Reason.* New York: Harper Collins.

Stivers C. 1991. The Politics of Public Health: The Dilemma of a Public Profession. In *Health Politics and Policy,* T. J. Litman and L. S. Robins, eds., New York: Delmar Publishers, Inc.

The Core Public Health Functions Steering Committee. 1994. *Public Health in America Statement.* Washington, D.C.: DHHS.

Turnock BJ, and Handler A. 1995. The 10 Public Health Practices vs. the 10 Public Health Services: A Clarification. Letter to the Editor. *American Journal of Public Health.* 85:1295–1296.

56

University of Illinois. 1994. Reinventing Public Health. *Leadership in Public Health* 3(3):1–36.

Vivier PM, Guyer B, and Hughart N. 1994. *Childhood Immunization Policy in the United States: An Historical Review (1962–1994).* Baltimore, Md.: Department of Maternal and Child Health, Johns Hopkins School of Hygiene and Public Health.

Washington Post series, January 28, 29, 31, and February 1 and 4, 1996. Based on *Washington Post*/Kaiser Family Foundation/Harvard University Survey Project, Why Don't Americans Trust the Government?

Washington State Department of Health. 1994. *Public Health Improvement Plan.* Olympia: Washington State Department of Health.

Woods DR, and Mason DD. 1992. Six Areas Lead National Early Immunization Drive. *Public Health Reports* 107(3):252–256.

Yates D. 1977. *The Ungovernable City: The Politics of Urban Problems and Policy Making.* Cambridge, Mass.: MIT Press.

Appendix A

Arnold and Mabel Beckman Center
Irvine, California

October 27, 1995

AGENDA

8:45–12:00 noon	**MORNING SESSION** *Stuart Bondurant, M.D., cochair*
8:45–9:00 a.m.	Welcome and Introductions
9:00–10:00 a.m	Goals of the Roundtable: What do we want to accomplish this year?
10:00–11:00 a.m.	Overview of *The Future of Public Health* *Hugh Tilson, M.D., Dr.P.H., cochair* *Edward Baker, M.D., Director, CDC Public Health* *Practice Program Office*
11:00–11:45 a.m.	Future of Public Health: Survey of Health Departments *F. Douglas Scutchfield, M.D., Visiting Scholar, Kaiser* *Permanente*

11:45–12:00 noon   Update on the APHA Session
                     Cynthia Abel, Program Officer

12:00–1:00 p.m.   Lunch

1:00–5:30 p.m.   **AFTERNOON SESSION**
                     Hugh Tilson, M.D., Dr.P.H., cochair

1:00–2:00 p.m.   California Medi-Cal Managed Care Program
                     *James G. Haughton, M.D., M.P.H., Senior Health
                       Services Policy Advisor, Los Angeles County
                       Department of Health Services
                     Ingrid Lamirault, Director, Planning and Policy
                       Development*

2:00–4:00 p.m.   Related Public Health Activities
                     Centers for Disease Control and Prevention
                     *David Satcher, M.D., Director, CDC
                     Edward Baker, M.D., Director, CDC Public Practice
                       Program Office*

                     Public Health Functions Project
                     Data/performance measurement for population health
                     Roz Lasker, M.D., New York Academy of Medicine

                     Expenditures, Workforce, Communications and
                       Community Planning
                     *Kristine M. Gebbie, R.N., Dr.P.H., F.A.A.N., Columbia
                       University School of Nursing*

                     Practice Guidelines
                     Edward Baker, M.D.

                     **The Robert Wood Johnson Foundation: Initiative on
                     Public Health Infrastructure**
                     *Nancy Kaufman, R.N., M.S., Vice President, The Robert
                       Wood Johnson Foundation*

                     The Kellogg Foundation
                     Thomas Bruce, M.D., Program Director

American Medical Association
James Allen, M.D., Director of Public Activities

Milbank Fund Project on Leadership in Public Health
Edward Baker, M.D.

IOM Committee on Using Performance Monitoring to Improve Community Health
John Lumpkin, M.D., M.P.H. (Committee Member)

The Linkages Council
Hugh Tilson, M.D., Dr.P.H.

Other Activities: Roundtable members are encouraged to talk about activities not mentioned above.

4:00–5:30 p.m.   General Discussion: Objectives of the Roundtable, Topics for Future Meetings, and Dates for Future Meetings
Stuart Bondurant, M.D., cochair
Hugh Tilson, M.D., Dr.P.H., cochair

PARTICIPANTS

Cynthia Abel
Program Officer
Institute of Medicine
Washington, DC

James Allen, M.D., M.P.H.
Vice President, Group on Science
  Technology and Public Health
American Medical Association
Chicago

Charles F. Bacon
Special Project Officer
Centers for Disease Control and
  Prevention
Atlanta
Edward L. Baker, M.D.

Director, Public Health Practice
  Program Office
Centers for Disease Control and
  Prevention
Atlanta

Steve Boedigheimer, M.M.
Deputy Director, Division of Public
  Health
Delaware Health and Social
  Services
Dover

Stuart Bondurant, M.D., *cochair*
Director, Center for Urban
 Epidemiologic Studies
New York Academy of Medicine
New York City

E. Richard Brown, Ph.D.
Professor of Public Health
School of Public Health and
Director, Center for Health Policy
 Research
University of California, Los
 Angeles

Thomas A. Bruce, M.D.
Program Director
W.K. Kellogg Foundation
Battle Creek, MI

Kristine M. Gebbie, R.N., Dr.P.H.,
 F.A.A.N.
Assistant Professor of Nursing
Columbia University School of
 Nursing
New York City

Margaret A. Hamburg, M.D.
(By conference call)
Health Commissioner
New York City Department of
 Health
New York City

James G. Haughton, M.D., M.P.H.
Senior Health Services Policy
 Advisor
County of Los Angeles
Department of Health Services
Los Angeles

Nancy Kaufman, R.N., M.S.
Vice President
The Robert Wood Johnson
 Foundation
Princeton, NJ

Ingrid Lamirault
Director, Planning and Policy
 Development
County of Los Angeles
Department of Health Services
Los Angeles

Roz Lasker, M.D.
Director, Division of Public Health
New York Academy of Medicine
New York City

John Lumpkin, M.D., M.P.H.
Director
Illinois Department of Public
 Health
Springfield

Charles Mahan, M.D.
Dean, College of Public Health
University of South Florida
College of Public Health

Kathy Newman, R.N., M.P.H.
Director, Barron County Public
 Health Nursing Service
Barron, WI

Robert Pestronk, M.P.H.
Health Officer
Genesee County Health
 Department
Flint, MI

David Satcher, M.D., Ph.D.
Director
Centers for Disease Control and
  Prevention
Atlanta

F. Douglas Scutchfield, M.D.
Visiting Scholar
Kaiser Permanente
Oakland, CA

Michael A. Stoto, Ph.D.
Director, Division of Health
  Promotion and Disease Prevention
Institute of Medicine
Washington, DC

Donna D. Thompson
Division Assistant
Institute of Medicine
Washington, DC

Hugh H. Tilson, M.D., Dr.P.H.,
  cochair
Vice President and Worldwide
  Director
Epidemiology Surveillance and
  Policy Research
Glaxo Wellcome Company
Research Triangle Park, NC

Robert B. Wallace, M.D.
Head, Department of Preventive
  Medicine and Environmental
  Health
University of Iowa

Martin Wasserman, M.D., J.D.
Secretary
Health and Mental Hygiene
  Department
State of Maryland
Baltimore

National Academy of Sciences
INSTITUTE OF MEDICINE

PUBLIC HEALTH ROUNDTABLE
APHA Session
San Diego, California
October 31, 1995

SUMMARY MINUTES

Introduction—Hugh Tilson, M.D., Dr. P.H.

Dr. Tilson introduced himself and outlined the format of the session and noted that speakers were selected from a variety of public health organizations and invited to prepare a short presentation in advance. Individuals who were asked to speak have reputations as visionaries who have the ability to look forward, but who are also aware of the realities of working in the public health field.

Presentations

Lead Abatement

■ **Lloyd Novick, M.D., SUNY School of Public Health, Linkages Council Chair**

Problems faced by different sectors of public health are similar, but standardized approaches to solving those problems are lacking. The Linkages Council is involved in evaluating the utility of public health guidelines in public health practice. However, there are difficulties associated with the development of standardized guidelines. For instance, differences between communities in terms of population and resources make it questionable whether the same guideline could provide optimal guidance to all communities. The Kellogg Foundation provided the Linkages Council with a grant to examine the usefulness of public health guidelines. Expert panels comprised of public health practitioners from state and local health departments, as well as the public health and clinical sectors, were convened to look at different areas of public health and review all relevant literature. One panel is looking at the usefulness of testing children for lead poisoning. A guideline would need to recommend whether all children in a community should be tested or whether limited resources should be focused on testing only low-income children, who are more likely to be exposed. The Linkages Council is presently working with the Public Health Service and the CDC with the intent of selecting two important public health topics and developing guidelines for them. The Public Health Service is also in the process of convening its own task force to examine the feasibility of guidelines.

■ Thomas Schlenker, M.D., Salt Lake City-County Health Department

Recent research has determined that low-level lead exposure can be harmful to young children and has helped to redefine childhood lead poisoning as a medical and social issue. In 1988 the CDC established a lead poisoning section to focus on issues related to childhood lead poisoning. Organizations such as the Alliance to End Childhood Lead Poisoning and the National Center for Lead-Safe Housing are collaborating with the CDC to define and combat the issue on a national level. However, some clinicians who treat young children never see lead poisoning in their patients, while others think they see it everywhere. There is also ongoing debate over whether the CDC's current danger level for lead exposure in young children of 10 μg/dcl is accurate. While the lead problem is well-defined nationally, Dr. Schlenker feels that the problem needs to be solved on a local level. It is the responsibility of local health departments to convince the medical community that lead poisoning is a problem that must be addressed. To achieve a greater awareness of lead issues, health departments need to collaborate with each other, the medical community, government agencies, and others, such as the construction and housing industries. Local health departments also need to collect data on blood lead levels in the populations they serve. In communities where blood lead levels have been monitored, the resulting data have been a sufficient basis for the development of lead-related programs.

STDs: Prevention and Control

■ Ellen Gursky, M.D., Department of Health, Trenton NJ

In New Jersey, the rates of syphilis and gonorrhea have decreased in recent years while the rate of HIV infection has leveled off. However, these trends are disproportionately distributed, in that rates remain very high in urban minority adolescent populations. Twenty-five percent of the patients in New Jersey STD clinics are adolescents. These facts illustrate the need for ongoing surveillance of STD morbidity. STD surveillance and prevention is handled mainly by state and local health departments, many of which receive state funding. As increasing numbers of patients are absorbed into managed care organizations and Medicaid managed care, surveillance of STDs and assurance of prevention activities, historically a key role of health departments, may become more challenged. In, addition, appropriate and timely treatment of STDs and epidemiologic follow-up may become compromised outside a public health system. On a national level, the surveillance of STDs and development of effective prevention programs will require the assurances of interconnected and standardized electronic information systems between managed care and public health systems.

■ Kathleen E. Toomey, M.D., M.P.H., Georgia Department of Human Resources

STD control programs in Georgia had remained stagnant over the past 50 years, until recently. Under the old system, Georgia had one of the highest rates of gonorrhea infection in the nation. The lack of standardization in reporting and poor data management under the old system made interpretation of gonorrhea data difficult. Improved communication both within different departments in the health department and among the health department, the medical community, and the local community, along with better data management, is essential for control of STDs. Better monitoring of infection rates for STDs could be used as a tool to focus resources. For example, 75% of the syphilis cases in Georgia are found in 25 counties, and prevention and control programs for STDs could be concentrated in those counties. The majority of women who delivered infants with congenital syphilis actually had received prenatal care and had been tested for syphilis. These women remained untreated because results of positive serologic tests for syphilis were not appropriately communicated among the various agencies providing care. State and local public health agencies need to play a more active role in the coordination and communication among all health care providers to successfully reduce this and other preventable STD complications.

■ Josh Lipsman, M.D., Alexandria Health Department

Dr. Lipsman outlined the services of the Alexandria, Virginia, Health Department. In Virginia, the local health department is a field office of the state health department, funded both by the city and the state. Services include family planning, administration of the WIC program, STD services and clinics, and full health clinics. The STD clinics are held three times a week on a walk-in basis. They are staffed by a different physician from the local community in rotation. To date in 1995, there have been approximately 2,000 visits to STD clinics in the Alexandria area. STD specialists interview each priority STD and HIV case and report each case to the state health department. If an individual from the Alexandria area is diagnosed with an STD in another part of Virginia, it is reported to the Alexandria health department, which takes responsibility for following the case. While Virginia's system for tracking and treating STD cases works well, it could be made more cost effective. Some of the tasks performed by physicians in the clinics could be reassigned. Nurses could be trained to collect specimens. Patients could be treated with a single-dose chlamydia treatment, which is more expensive than the standard treatment, but also more effective. Many patients also seek primary care services from the STD clinics. These patients are referred elsewhere. More community involvement and education regarding STD programs is essential. The overall trend in Alexandria and in Virginia has been toward a decrease in STDs over the past four years. The decrease in STDs may be attributable to education programs in the state and tracking of STDs by local health departments.

Family Violence

■ Elizabeth McLoughlin, So.D., San Francisco General Hospital

To date, family violence issues have been addressed for the most part not by the traditional public health system, but by the women's movement, shelters, and grassroots efforts. It has been determined that *Healthy People 2000* objectives related to family violence (reduction of physical abuse to 27/10,000 couples and reduction in the number of battered women to less than 10%) are not being met.

It is difficult to develop statistics on family violence since the system for collecting incidence data on spousal abuse and violence against women is not very effective. Much abuse still goes unreported to anyone outside the family. In order to define the problem it is necessary to collect data on the incidence of family violence and establish some baseline statistics. To this end, the CDC recently established a task force to develop strategies for surveillance of family violence. The public health sector needs to get more involved in family violence issues in general. In the past, the public health sector has assisted women's organizations and others who have taken the lead in combating family violence, but public health should now take a leadership role. Some strategies for reducing family violence include educating judges about family violence; working with immigrant women, who traditionally have had a significant problem with spousal abuse; and working to change societal norms so that family abuse becomes unacceptable.

■ Alex Kelter, M.D., California Department of Health Services

Definitions of family violence differ from agency to agency and state to state. In California, data on family violence is collected separately from data on other forms of violence. One obstacle to collecting data on family violence is the public perception that reporting of family violence has little benefit and may incur high risk. As with other public health issues, health departments need to form partnerships with the community, other agencies and the medical community. The increase in managed care organizations is creating new challenges for health departments. Health departments need to think of incentives to get managed care organizations to report public health problems, such as domestic violence. Dr. Kelter suggested that health departments take the lead in violence prevention in their communities. However, better surveillance and research into family violence issues is needed to understand the depth of the problem. For example, it is not known if women who use shelters to escape abusive spouses have better outcomes than those who do not. Domestic violence prevention programs also need to be focused on men, not just women.

■ Desmond Runyan, M.D., University of North Carolina

Several years ago there was considerable focus on child abuse issues in the public health field. In recent years, however, the focus has shifted from child abuse to family violence. Efforts to assess the extent of the child abuse problem in the United States have been hampered by a lack of uniformity in data collection among different states, leading to difficulty in pooling data, and the lack of a uniformly accepted definition of child abuse. Legislation recently approved by the House of Representatives would have eradicated the National Center for Child Abuse and Neglect and sent the money to the states instead. This action by the House further impedes collection of data on child abuse as it will take some time for the states to set up programs. In response to concerns over child abuse, North Carolina initiated the North Carolina Child Abuse Evaluation Program. This program enlists community physicians and provides them with continuing education related to the identification and prevention of child abuse. The State of North Carolina pays for all education and exams for participating physicians. Most physicians who participate are dedicated to the program and have formed a network in the state. However, the educational programs focus mainly on physical abuse; as a result, physicians still lack knowledge about the sexual abuse of children.

Appendix B

Conference Room 2004 , 1055 Thomas Jefferson Street, N.W.
Washington, DC

February 22, 1996

AGENDA

Workshop on Public Health and Managed Care

8:30 a.m.	Introduction of the Public Health Roundtable Members and Recap of First Roundtable Meeting (October 1995) *Stuart Bondurant and Hugh Tilson, cochairs*
8:45 a.m.	Welcome to the Institute of Medicine *Kenneth I. Shine, IOM President*
9:00 a.m.	IOM Activities Related to Public Health and Managed Care
	IOM Board on Health Promotion and Disease Prevention: Workshop on the Impact of Medicaid Managed Care on Children, *Hugh Tilson*

IOM Committee on Using Performance Monitoring to
Improve Community Health, *Kristine Gebbie*

IOM Committee on the Prevention and Control of STDs,
Richard Brown

9:30 a.m.–12:30 p.m.	Public Health and Managed Care: Shared Responsibilities

Perspectives of Public Health Agencies

9:30 a.m.   State health department perspective
Anne Barry, Commissioner of Health, Minnesota
David Smith, Commissioner of Health, Texas

10:30 a.m.   Local health department perspective
Paul Simms, Deputy Director, Department of Health
Services, County of San Diego

11:00 a.m.   BREAK

11:15 a.m.   Perspectives of Managed Care Organizations

For-profit HMO perspective
Sandy Harmon-Weiss, Medical Director, U.S. Healthcare

Not-for-profit HMO perspective
William Beery, Director, Center for Health Promotion,
Group Health Cooperative of Puget Sound, Seattle

12:30 p.m.   LUNCH

1:30–5:45 p.m.   Roundtable Discussion on Shared Responsibilities and
Building Partnerships

Between Public Health Departments and Managed Care
Organizations

PARTICIPANTS

Cynthia Abel
Program Officer
Institute of Medicine
Washington, DC

Rhoda Abrams
Health Resources and Services
  Administration
Bureau of Primary Health Care
Bethesda, MD

Jim Allen, M.D., M.P.H.
Vice President, Group on Science
  Technology and Public Health
American Medical Association
Chicago

Charles F. Bacon
Special Project Officer
Centers for Disease Control and
  Prevention
Atlanta

Edward L. Baker, M.D.
Director, Public Health Practice
  Program Office
Centers for Disease Control and
  Prevention
Atlanta

Anne M. Barry, J.D., M.P.H.
Commissioner of Health
Minnesota Department of Health
Minneapolis

Michael Barry
Public Health Foundation
Washington, DC

William Beery, M.P.H.
Director
Center for Health Promotion
Group Health Cooperative of Puget
  Sound
Seattle, WA

Cheryl A. Beversdorf, R.N., M.H.S.
Executive Vice-President
Association of State and Territorial
  Health Officials
Washington, DC

Steve Boedigheimer, M.M.
Deputy Director, Division of Public
  Health
Delaware Health and Social
  Services
Dover

Stuart Bondurant, M.D., *cochair*
Director, Center for Urban
  Epidemiologic Studies
New York Academy of Medicine
New York City

Jo Ivey Boufford, M.D.
Principal Deputy Assistant Secretary
  for Health
U.S. Public Health Service
Department of Health and Human
  Services
Washington, DC

E. Richard Brown, Ph.D.
Professor of Public Health
School of Public Health and
Director, Center for Health Policy
  Research
University of California, Los Angeles

Thomas A. Bruce
Program Director
W.K. Kellogg Foundation
Little Rock, AR

Jackie L. Bryan, R.N., M.S.
Director of Health Policy
Association of State and Territorial
  Health Officials
Washington, DC

Barbara Calkins, M.A.
Executive Director
Association of Teachers of Preventive
  Medicine
Washington, DC

D.W. Chen, M.D.
Health Resources and Services
  Administration
Bureau of Health Professions
Rockville, MD

Jordon J. Cohen, M.D.
President
Association of American Medical
  Colleges
Washington, DC

Jane Durch, M.S.
Senior Program Officer
Institute of Medicine
Washington, DC

Margo Edmunds, Ph.D.
Senior Program Officer
Institute of Medicine
Washington, DC

Tom Eng, V.M.D., M.P.H.
Senior Program Officer
Institute of Medicine
Washington, DC

Caswell A. Evans, Jr., D.D.S., M.P.H.
Assistant Director of Health Services
Director, Public Health Programs and
  Services
County of Los Angeles
Department of Health Services
Los Angeles

Claude Earl Fox, M.D., M.P.H.
Deputy Assistant Secretary for Health
Director, Office of Disease
  Prevention and Health Promotion
Department of Health and Human
  Services
Washington, DC

Carol Galaty
Health Resources and Services
  Administration
Maternal and Child Health Bureau
Rockville, MD

Kristine M. Gebbie, R.N., Dr.P.H.,
  F.A.A.N.
Assistant Professor of Nursing
Columbia University School of
  Nursing

Michael K. Gemmell, C.A.E.
Executive Director
Association of Schools of Public
 Health
Washington, DC

Liza Greenberg
Group Health Association of
 America
Washington, DC

Margaret A. Hamburg, M.D.
Health Commissioner
New York City Department of
 Health
New York City

Karen Ignagni
President and CEO
Group Health Association of
 America
Washington, DC

Nancy Kaufman, R.N., M.S.
Vice President
The Robert Wood Johnson
 Foundation
Princeton, NJ

Hazel K. Keimowitz, M.A.
Executive Director
American College of Preventive
 Medicine
Washington, DC

Roz Lasker, M.D.
Director, Division of Public Health
New York Academy of Medicine
New York City

John Lumpkin, M.D., M.P.H.
Director
Illinois Department of Public Health
Springfield

Charles Mahan, M.D.
Dean, College of Public Health
University of South Florida

Katherine Marconi
Health Resources and Services
 Administration
Bureau of Health and Development
Rockville, MD

Kathy Newman, R.N., M.P.H.
Director
Barron County Health Department
Barron, WI

Rebecca Parkins, Ph.D., M.P.H.
Director, Scientific Professions and
 Section Affairs
American Public Health Association
Washington, DC

Iris Posner
Health Resources and Services
 Administration
Bureau of Health and Development
Rockville, MD

Robert Pestronk, M.P.H.
Health Officer
Genesee County Health Department
Flint, MI

Nancy Rawding, M.P.H.
Executive Director
National Association of County and
 City Health Officials
Washington, DC

Jud Richland
Executive Director
Partnership for Prevention
Washington, DC

Alex Ross, Sc.D.
Public Health Analyst
Office of Public Health Practice
Health Resources and Services
 Administration
Rockville, MD

David Satcher, M.D., Ph.D.
Director
Centers for Disease Control and
 Prevention
Atlanta

Kenneth I. Shine, M.D.
President
Institute of Medicine
Washington, DC

Paul Simms, M.P.H.
Deputy Director
Department of Community Health
 Services
County of San Diego
San Diego

David Smith, M.D.
Commissioner of Health
Texas Department of Health
Austin

Paul Stange, M.P.H.
Public Health Consultant
Centers for Disease Control and
 Prevention
Atlanta

Michael A. Stoto, Ph.D.
Director, Division of Health
 Promotion and Disease Prevention
Institute of Medicine
Washington, DC

Ciro Sumaya, M.D.
Administrator
Health Resources and Services
 Administration
Rockville, MD

Donna D. Thompson
Division Assistant
Institute of Medicine
Washington, DC

Hugh H. Tilson, M.D., Dr.P.H.,
 cochair
Vice President and Worldwide
 Director
Epidemiology Surveillance and
 Policy Research
Glaxo Wellcome Company
Research Triangle Park, NC

Robert B. Wallace, M.D.
Head, Department of Preventive
 Medicine and Environmental
 Health
University of Iowa

Martin Wasserman, M.D., J.D.
Secretary
Health and Mental Hygiene
  Department
State of Maryland
Baltimore

Sandy Harmon-Weiss, M.D.
Senior Vice President and Medical
  Director
U.S. Healthcare
Blue Bell, PA

Peter Van Dyke, M.D.
Chief Medical Officer
Health Resources and Services
  Administration
Maternal and Child Health Bureau
Rockville, MD

Herbert F. Young, M.D.
Director, Activities Division
American Academy of Family
  Physicians
Kansas City, MO

Appendix C

PUBLIC HEALTH ROUNDTABLE
Centers for Disease Control and Prevention
Building 16, Conference Room 1107
Atlanta

June 27, 1996

AGENDA

Workshop on Public Health and Public Policy

8:45 a.m.	Welcome to the Centers for Disease Control and Prevention *David Satcher, Director*
9:00 a.m.	Opening Remarks *Stuart Bondurant and Hugh Tilson, cochairs*
9:15–9:45 a.m.	Public Trust and Confidence in Government: How Can Governmental Agencies Respond to Public Mistrust of Government *Todd LaPorte, University of California at Berkeley*

9:45 a.m.–12:45 p.m.   Panel Session I: Public Health in the Community
                       Robert Pestronk, Moderator

                       Panel Members:
                       Liane Levetan, Chief Executive Officer, Dekalb County
                       Paul Wiesner, Director of DeKalb County Health
                           Department.
                       Steve Margolis, Assistant Director for Special Projects,
                           Division of Public Health for Georgia
                       Jo Ann Thomas, Director, Life Skills Center
                       J. Frederick Agel, Chairman, DeKalb Board of Health
                       Yvonne Lewis, Program Coordinator, Flint and Vicinity
                           Action Community Economic Development, Inc.

                       Respondent:
                       Arden Miller, Professor Emeritus of Maternal and Child
                           Health, University of North Carolina, Chapel Hill

12:45–2:00 p.m.   **LUNCH**

2:00–5:00 p.m.   Panel Session II: The Role of State Government in Public
                           Health
                       Martin Wasserman, Moderator

                       Speaker (to frame the issues of the panel session):
                       Randy Desonia, Director of Policy Studies, Health Policy

                       Panel members:
                       Patrick Meehan, Director, Georgia Division of Public
                           Health
                       Senator Nadine Thomas, Vice Chairman, Committee on
                           Health and Human Services, Georgia Senate
                       Lawrence Sanders, Medical Director for Managed Care,
                           Grady Health System
                       Joyce Essien, Director, Center for Public Health
                           Prevention, Emory University School of Public Health

5:00 p.m.   Concluding Remarks
                       Stuart Bondurant and Hugh Tilson, cochairs

PARTICIPANTS

Cynthia Abel
Program Officer
Institute of Medicine
Washington, DC

J. Frederick Agel
President, DeKalb County Local
  Board of Health
Southeast Regional Trustee of the
  Executive Board of the
  Association of Local Boards of
  Health
Atlanta

Charles F. Bacon
Special Project Officer
Centers for Disease Control and
  Prevention
Atlanta

Edward L. Baker, M.D.
Director, Public Health Practice
  Program Office
Centers for Disease Control and
  Prevention
Atlanta

Steve Boedigheimer, M.M.
Deputy Director, Division of Public
  Health
Delaware Health and Social
  Services
Dover

Stuart Bondurant, M.D., *cochair*
Director, Center for Urban
Epidemiologic Studies
New York Academy of Medicine
New York City

E. Richard Brown, Ph.D.
Professor of Public Health
School of Public Health, and
Director, Center for Health Policy
  Research
University of California, Los
  Angeles

Thomas A. Bruce, M.D.
Program Director
W.K. Kellogg Foundation
Little Rock, AR

Joe H. Davis, M.D., M.P.H.
Director
International Health Program
  Office
Centers for Disease Control and
  Prevention
Atlanta

Randy Desonia
Director of Policy Studies
Health Policy Division
National Governors' Association
Washington, DC

Anne Dievler, Ph.D.
Interim Director of Masters of
  Health Science Program in Health
  Policy
School of Hygiene and Public
  Health
Johns Hopkins University

Joyce Essien, M.D., M.B.A.
Director, Center for Public Health
  Prevention
Rollins School of Public Health
  Practice
Emory University

Caswell A. Evans, Jr., D.D.S.,
  M.P.H.
Assistant Director of Health
  Services
Director, Public Health Programs
  and Services
County of Los Angeles
Department of Health Services
Los Angeles

Claude Earl Fox, M.D., M.P.H.
Deputy Assistant Secretary for
  Health
Director, Office of Disease
  Prevention and Health Promotion
Department of Health and Human
  Services
Washington, DC

Kristine M. Gebbie, R.N., Dr.P.H.,
  F.A.A.N.
Assistant Professor of Nursing
Columbia University School of
  Nursing

Liza Greenberg
American Association of Health
  Plans
Washington, DC

Margaret A. Hamburg, M.D.
Health Commissioner
New York City Department of
  Health
New York City

James M. Hughes, M.D.
Director
National Center for Infectious
  Diseases
Centers for Disease Control and
  Prevention
Atlanta

Barry L. Johnson, Ph.D.
Assistant Administrator
Agency for Toxic Substances and
  Disease Registry
Atlanta

Todd LaPorte
Professor, Department of Political
  Sciences
University of California at
  Berkeley

Roz Lasker, M.D.
(by conference call)
Director, Division of Public Health
New York Academy of Medicine
New York City

Liane Levetan
Chief Executive Officer
DeKalb County Government
Decatur

Yvonne Lewis
Program Coordinator
Flint and Vicinity Action
  Community Economic
  Development, Inc. (FACED)
Flint, MI

Doug Lloyd, M.D., M.PH.
Associate Administrator, Public
  Health Practice
Health Resources and Services
  Administration
Rockville, MD

John Lumpkin, M.D., M.P.H.
Director
Illinois Department of Public
  Health
Springfield

Charles Mahan, M.D.
Dean, College of Public Health
University of South Florida

Steven Margolis, Ph.D.
Assistant Director for Special
  Projects
Division of Public Health
Atlanta

Patrick J. Meehan, M.D.
Director
Division of Public Health
Atlanta

C. Arden Miller, M.D.
Professor Emeritus of Maternal and
  Child Health
School of Public Health
Department of Maternal and Child
  Health
University of North Carolina,
  Chapel Hill

Kathy Newman, R.N., M.P.H.
Director, Barron County Health
  Department
Barron, WI

Walter A. Orenstein, M.D.
Director
National Immunization Program
Centers for Disease Control and
  Prevention
Atlanta

Robert Pestronk, M.P.H.
Health Officer
Genesee County Health
  Department
Flint, MI

Mark L. Rosenberg, M.D., M.P.P.
Director
National Center for Injury
  Prevention and Control
Centers for Disease Control and
  Prevention
Atlanta

Linda Rosenstock, M.D., M.P.H.
Director
National Institute for Occupational
  Safety and Health
Washington, DC

Lawrence Sanders M.D.
Medical Director for Managed
  Care
Grady Health System
Atlanta

David Satcher, M.D., Ph.D.
Director
Centers for Disease Control and
  Prevention
Atlanta

Tonia Smith
Computer Secretary
Atlanta

Dixie E. Snider, Jr., M.D., M.P.H.
Associate Director for Science
Centers for Disease Control and
  Prevention
Atlanta

Michael A. Stoto, Ph.D.
Director, Division of Health
  Promotion and Disease
  Prevention
Institute of Medicine
Washington, DC

Ciro Sumaya, M.D.
Administrator
Health Resources and Services
  Administration
Rockville, MD

Jo Ann Thomas
Director
Life Skills Center
Marietta

Senator Nadine Thomas
Georgia State Senate
Atlanta

Donna Thompson
Division Assistant
Institute of Medicine
Washington, DC

Hugh H. Tilson, M.D., Dr.P.H.,
  cochair
Vice President and Worldwide
  Director
Epidemiology Surveillance and
  Policy Research
Glaxo Wellcome Company
Research Triangle Park, NC

Cynthia Tucker
Public Health Advisor
Georgia Senate Committee on
  Health and Human Services
Atlanta

Vaughn Upshaw, M.P.H.
Chairperson
Chattham County Board of Health
Pittsboro, NC

Robert B. Wallace, M.D.
Head, Department of Preventive
  Medicine and Environmental
  Health
University of Iowa

Martin Wasserman, M.D., J.D.
Secretary
Health and Mental Hygiene
  Department
State of Maryland

Paul J. Wiesner, M.D.
Director
DeKalb County Board of Health
Decatur

David Williamson
Acting Director
Division of Diabetes Translation
National Center for Chronic
   Disease Prevention and Health
   Promotion
Centers for Disease Control and
   Prevention
Atlanta